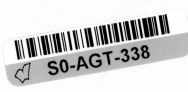

Neurobiology for Clinical Social Work

Neurobiology for Clinical Social Work

Theory and Practice

Jeffrey S. Applegate

Janet R. Shapiro

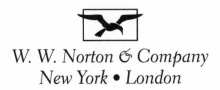

W. W. Norton & Company
New York • London

Production Manager: Leeann Graham
Manufacturing by Haddon Craftsmen
Composition by Bytheway

Library of Congress Cataloging-in-Publication Data

Applegate, Jeffrey S.
Neurobiology for clinical social work : theory and practice / Jeffrey S. Applegate,
Janet R. Shapiro.
p.   cm.
"A Norton professional book."
Includes bibliographical references and index.
ISBN 0-393-70420-3
1. Neurobiology.   2. Neuropsychology.   3. Clinical sociology.   I. Shapiro, Janet R.
II. Title.

QP355.2.A65 2005
612.8—dc22   2005045082

W. W. Norton & Company, Inc., 500 Fifth Avenue, New York, N.Y. 10110
www.wwnorton.com

W. W. Norton & Company Ltd., Castle House, 75/76 Wells St., London W1T 3QT

1   3   5   7   9   0   8   6   4   2

CONTENTS

ACKNOWLEDGMENTS

WE GRATEFULLY acknowledge the assistance of many people in the preparation of this book. We would like to thank our colleagues at Bryn Mawr College for their support. In particular, the sabbatical we each received was critical to our ability to engage new ideas. We would also like to thank our editor at Norton Professional Books, Deborah Malmud, and her associate, Michael McGandy, for their careful attention to detail, their understanding of our perspective, and their consistent encouragement. Finally, we are grateful to our families for their ongoing patience and support.

INTRODUCTION

OUR PURPOSE IN WRITING this book is to inform clinical social workers and social work educators about new findings from research on the neurobiology of attachment and their implications for knowledge building and clinical practice. These findings contribute to the understanding of how individuals regulate emotion and its affective expression, termed *affect regulation*. There is increasing consensus among scholars of human development that this self-regulatory capacity is central to well-being throughout the lifespan, and that affect dysregulation is a central risk factor in a wide range of psychosocial difficulties.

The last 15 years have produced a virtual explosion of research on the neurobiology of attachment and the ways in which modes of affect regulation play a key role in determining the structure and function of the developing brain and mind. Psychoanalytically informed scholars have taken leadership in reporting these findings in terms of their relevance for clinical theory and practice. Although the resulting literature comprises an impressive compendium, it is aimed primarily toward a psychoanalytic audience. To date no book intended for social workers exists; yet, by virtue of their work with at-risk children and families whose capacity for affect regulation is challenged by such factors as poverty, environmental deprivation, oppression, and societal violence, social workers occupy a unique position from which to employ this new knowledge in prevention and intervention.

The research we report offers new insights about the crucial role that relationships play in human development and in professional helping efforts. By describing the specific biopsychosocial processes that constitute the relationship, we hope to contribute to longstanding inquiry of the social work field into its mysteries.

RELATIONSHIP: THE ELUSIVE CONCEPT

From its inception, the social work profession has placed the helping relationship at the center of its theorizing and practice. Enduringly focused on the person-in-environment in the wide variety of settings and modalities in which they practice, social workers across the decades have extolled the importance of the web of relationships in their clients' lives and the mutative power of the therapeutic relationship in their work with these clients. Whether working with individuals, families, groups, or communities, social workers have long recognized that it is the client's *experience* of the helping relationship, as much as or more than the worker's resource provision, clever interpretations, or other technical interventions, that facilitates change.

Although implicit in the writing of late 19th- and early 20th-century social work scholars, the earliest use of the term *relationship* in the professional literature can be traced to Virginia Robinson's book, *A Changing Psychology in Social Casework*, published in 1930 (as cited in Biestek, 1957). Since then, scores of social work scholars have worked toward a definition of this intuitively accessible but conceptually elusive term. Authors have cited warmth, caring, acceptance, genuineness, a nonjudgmental attitude, responsiveness, empathy, attentiveness, support, concern, and understanding as core components of helpful relationships. The relationship has been characterized as the "heart" of the helping process (Perlman, 1979) and "the soul of [social] casework" (Biestek, 1957). Such efforts to convey the essence of relationship notwithstanding, the concept continues to elude efforts to capture in words its complexity and the skill it takes to employ it effectively.

PSYCHOANALYTIC PERSPECTIVES ON THE RELATIONSHIP

Early on, social workers began to look beyond their own professional boundaries for assistance in articulating the central role of the relationship in their work. Beginning in the 1920s, many social workers engaged in direct practice discovered in Freud's psychoanalytic theory a more thoroughly elaborated vocabulary with which to describe their practice. Terms such as *transference, countertransference,* and *resistance* offered new language for understanding relationship dynamics. With the ascendancy of ego psychology in the 1930s, social workers found in such concepts as ego functions, defense, and adaptation additional conceptual tools for describing the relational aspects of their work. Ego psychology opened a path for further exploration of the nontransferential or "real" aspects of the relationship, captured in such terms as the working or therapeutic alliance (Brenner, 1979, as cited in Moore & Fine, 1990).

Yet neither classical drive theory nor ego psychology sufficiently explained what it is that makes the relationship *qua* relationship so influential. Beginning in the 1940s, clinical theorists in Great Britain and the United States began to elaborate a theory of object relations, effectively moving psychoanalysis from a one-person psychology based on a closed-system model of internal conflict, defense, and compromise formation to a two-person psychology focused on the relational dynamics between analyst and analysand (Greenberg & Mitchell, 1983). Object relations theorists put the relationship in the spotlight of their inquiry, offering social workers further refined concepts and language with which to describe their work with rigor, depth, and technical explication. Winnicott's (1965a) concept of ego relatedness and Bowlby's (1969) description of the dynamics of human attachment, for example, expanded the conceptual lens through which to view relationships and their mutative impact.

In the 1970s Heinz Kohut (1971, 1977) employed object relations theory as a base from which to launch his self psychology, focusing on such processes as empathy, mirroring, idealization of others, and twinship as aspects of relationship that are important developmentally and therapeutically. Both object relations theorists and self psychologists have emphasized the role of internalization in the development of interpersonal relatedness. Tracing this process to earliest development, they suggest that, during countless interactions between child and caregiver, caregiving functions are gradually taken in (i.e., internalized) by the child as templates for relational interactions throughout life—templates that will also shape how they experience and behave in therapeutic relationships.

Most recently, theorists of intersubjectivity have focused on the interplay of the inner lives and unique subjectivity of both parties—child and caregiver, client and clinician—in cocreating and sustaining adaptive relationships (Stolorow, Atwood, & Brandchaft, 1994), part of a broader metapsychology termed "relational theory" (Aron, 1996; Mitchell, 1988). Recognizing that social work has always been "relational," today's social work scholars are adding richly to the literature of this broader theoretical shift (see, e.g., Applegate & Bonovitz, 1995; Edward & Sanville, 1996; Elson, 1986; Goldstein, 2001; Saari, 2002; Sanville, 1991; Seinfeld, 1991). Many of these contributions illustrate the power of the supportive, sustaining, empathic qualities of the helping relationship referred to by Imre (1982) as "clinical caring."

Yet the questions remain: How, exactly, does the relationship do its work? How does the warmth, acceptance, genuineness, attentiveness, concern, responsiveness, and understanding conveyed by one person influence the well-being of another? Almost a half century ago, Perlman suggested that "relationship leaps from one person to the other at the moment when emotion moves between them" (1957, p. 65). This description seems almost mystical at first; but a second look reveals that it was prescient of current multidisciplinary research, which promises to offer all the helping professions exciting new tools for conceptualizing and making use of the relationship in their work.

NEW DIRECTIONS

A remarkable convergence of research findings has occurred from the study of attachment, developmental psychology, nonlinear dynamic systems theory, cognitive neuroscience, and neurobiology suggesting that, indeed, it is the movement of emotion between individuals that connects them in dynamic, reciprocal relationships. New conceptions of emotion suggest that its primary function is to coordinate processes in the mind with those of the body (Pally, 2000). Pally suggested that "emotion connects not only the mind of body of one individual but minds and bodies *between* individuals" (p. 74, italics in original). One reason that it may have been so difficult to articulate the dynamics of relationship is that the "leap" of emotion between people is increasingly believed to occur at a nonconscious, nonverbal level (Pally, 2000; Schore, 1994; Siegel, 1999).

Of course we are aware of certain emotions—joy, sadness, anger—and are able to put many feelings into words. Recent research suggests, however, that the conscious awareness and verbalization of emotion are merely the tip of the iceberg. Findings from this inquiry suggest that most emotion "moves" between people not in words but primarily in forms that may not be registered in conscious perception—facial expressions, gestures, postural changes, and such prosodic elements as tone, rhythm, and quality of speech. When one individual's nonverbal communication matches another's, the resulting synchrony "recreates inside that person the autonomic changes and body sensations associated with the other's emotional state. We may literally feel what another feels" (Pally, 2000, p. 97).

AFFECT REGULATION

The nonverbal expressions of emotion described above are typically referred to as "affective expressions" or simply "affect" (Siegel, 1999, p. 128). In this conceptualization, facial expressions, shifts in posture, and various gestures are outward expressions of internal feelings states. When two people who are interacting achieve moments of matching or mirroring each other's nonverbal expressions of subjectively experienced emotion, they are engaged in mutual "affect regulation" (Schore, 1994). The capacity for affect regulation is believed to be generated in the earliest interactions between infants and their caregivers. It is during the earliest "dance" of mutual affect regulation in the infant–caregiver dyad that modes of regulating intense emotions are learned and internalized by the infant in ways that shape the development of brain structure and function. In other words, modes of early affect regulation become "hard-wired" into neuronal structures that shape the individual's subsequent modes of relating throughout life.

Knowledge generated by the multidisciplinary study of affect regulation and its role in attachment offers a new conceptual window through which to view the development of emotionally meaningful relationships, including the clinical relationship. This knowledge adds conceptual rigor to social work's biopsychosocial conception of human behavior and offers new insights into ways in which the clinical process can enhance clients' capacity for affect regulation. Helping clients regulate the behavioral expression of feeling states is increasingly recognized as a crucial goal of social work helping efforts. Styles of affect regulation tend to be passed from one generation to the next (Crandall, Fitzgerald, & Whipple, 1997), and many families with whom social workers come into contact are at risk for affect dysregulation in ways that compromise their relational capacities. Children developing in these families are likely to internalize ways of handling strong emotions that place them at risk for later psychopathology (Bradley, 2000). Many of these children develop with impaired ability to sooth themselves, modulate states of intense emotional arousal, respond adaptively to over- or understimulation by caregivers, or regulate aggressive and sexual impulses. Later sequelae of these vulnerabilities include mood disturbances, personality disorders, maladaptive modes of reacting to stress, abusive behavior toward others, and substance abuse (which represents misdirected attempts at self-medicating internal distress).

BRAIN, MIND, AND EMOTION

During the 1990s, the "decade of the brain" (Gabbard, 1992), the study of emotion and its affective expression advanced dramatically in conjunction with the refinement of neuropsychology, electrophysiology, and various neuroimaging technologies. Researchers using these new tools have erased previous notions of a dichotomy between brain and mind. Today brain and mind are seen as being in constant synergistic, dynamic interaction, and, as a result, "all mental phenomena are assumed to be the result of biological activity of neuronal circuits of the brain" (Pally, 2000, p. 1). Predetermined genetic programming dominates the development of these circuits during gestation and for a few months postpartum. But from birth onward, the infant's experiences in the interpersonal environment play a major role in determining which connections become functionally active (Pally, 2000). As Siegel put it, "the mind develops at the interface of neurophysiological processes and interpersonal relationships" (1999, p. 21).

NEUROBIOLOGY AND CLINICAL PRACTICE:
THE QUESTION OF RELEVANCE

Sydney Pulver, a psychoanalyst, published an article titled "On the Astonishing Clinical Irrelevance of Neuroscience" (2003), in which he stressed the point that, although neuroscience has contributed significantly to psychoanalytic *theory*, to date little evidence has been provided that it has much new to add to clinical *technique*. It is likely that the same argument could be made about many current approaches that address people's problems in living. We believe, however, that even though neuroscience may not offer "new" techniques for these modes of intervention—and therefore may not be technically "astonishing"—it is, indeed, clinically relevant.

First, rather than offering radical new intervention techniques, recent research findings from the neurosciences appear to provide evidence that supports the efficacy of certain tried-and-true approaches. For example, Schore (2003b) reviewed research by Furmark and associates (2002) demonstrating that symptomatic improvement during cognitive–behavioral therapy for socially phobic clients is accompanied by increased blood flow to the area of the brain associated with affect regulation. Similarly, both Schore (2003b) and Cozolino (2002) cited another study by Schwartz and colleagues (1996) that demonstrated changes in brain metabolism following behavior modification for obsessive–compulsive disorder.

Schore suggested that, whatever the theoretical approach, it is the clinical relationship that "acts as a growth promoting environment that supports the experience-dependent maturation of the right brain, especially those areas that have connections with the subcortical limbic structures that mediate emotional arousal" (1994, p. 473). This formulation lends a biological dimension to the conclusion drawn from numerous studies that the helping relationship, rather than specific techniques, is the key mutative factor in therapeutic effectiveness. This relationship has been referred to as a facilitating partnership (Applegate & Bonovitz, 1995), a holding environment (Winnicott, 1965d), a growth-facilitating environment (Schore, 2003b), and an enriched environment (Cozolino,

2002). All these terms strive to capture the qualities of the interpersonal "space" of clinical intervention and its centrality to successful helping efforts.

As noted, from its inception the social work profession has emphasized the clinician–client relational matrix as the most potent element in promoting change in people and their environments. With the development of clinical social work as a specialty within the profession, its practitioners borrowed from psychodynamic, cognitive–behavioral, and systemic approaches in order to address the wide range of issues presented by clients in various settings. The skillful deployment of techniques associated with these approaches, however, has always depended on the overarching interpersonal skills of relationship development. More than adding new techniques to clinical social workers' repertoire, findings from neurobiology help them appreciate the biopsychosocial substrate of relational dynamics that serve as a context for effectively applying techniques they already use.

We argue, therefore, that social work is not looking for "astonishing" technical relevance. Rather, we believe that an acquaintance with neuroscientific findings can add rigorous conceptual support to something that has eluded clear explication: the power and empowering potential of the clinical relationship. Moreover, recent scholarship by Bradley (2000), Cozolino (2002), and Schore (2003b) may lead the way to challenging Pulver's (2003) assertion that neuroscience is clinically irrelevant. As we describe in the chapters to follow, their work attempts to explain the neurobiological basis for the way in which clinical intervention can enhance neural network integration and thereby enhance adaptive affect regulation.

Clearly, neurobiologically informed clinical work is an emerging field of practice. Our hope is that this book will stimulate clinical social workers to think about and apply some of the ideas we explicate. By virtue of their work in a wide array of settings with diverse populations, clinical social workers have a unique opportunity to join clinicians from other disciplines in exploring the practice implications of these this exciting new field of inquiry.

PLAN OF THE BOOK

Understanding the nature of this convergence of neurological and re-lational processes requires a basic knowledge of brain structure and func-tioning, memory, affect, and attachment, and the ways in which these phenomena shape, and are shaped by, intimate relationships with others through contingent communication and the mutual regulation of affect. To set the stage for this inquiry, in Chapter 1 we introduce fundamentals of brain structure, development, and functioning. This introduction is in-tended as a primer and proceeds from the assumption that many readers are relatively unfamiliar with the field of brain science. We focus our re-view on those aspects of the brain's development and function that are most useful in understanding affect regulation. In Chapter 2 we examine the neurobiology of memory; in Chapter 3, a neuropsychological con-ceptualization of affect. In these two chapters we focus on the manner in which memory and affect perform their organizational functions within and between minds.

In Chapter 4 we examine precursors to attachment that evolve during the earliest months of the infant's life, focusing on the way the caregiver helps "organize" the infant, and vice versa. In considering these early expressions of affect regulation, we use the conceptual lens of nonlinear dynamic sys-tems theory to consider the role of temperament and constitutional factors as additional variables that may influence the "goodness of fit" (Chess & Thomas, 1991) between infant and caregiver; and we examine possible ways in which these and other variables contribute to resilience or increase the vulnerability to risk factors.

In Chapter 5 we address attachment as an expression of more mature mutual affect regulation. Following a review of Bowlby's (1969) original theory and a description of attachment classifications, we explore, in turn, Mary Ainsworth's research on the Strange Situation (Ainsworth, Blehar, Waters, & Wall, 1978) and Mary Main's work on adult attachment styles (Main & Goldwyn, 1991). This review acts as a basis for considering the capacity for "mentalization" and its associated "reflective function" (Fon-agy, Gergely, Jurist, & Target, 2002), ideas that tie the capacity to intuit and become empathically attuned to the mental and emotional states of others to affect regulation.

In Chapter 6 we turn from theory to practice, beginning with examples of caregiving dyads at risk for affect dysregulation and its relational seque-lae. (Note that all case examples in the book are composites.) Examples include adolescent parents and their children, children with a depressed parent, and children of parents who abuse substances. In Chapter 7 we consider infant mental health interventions as prevention efforts designed to identify early expressions of affect dysregulation in such families and re-view strategies for helping them reestablish regulation. We pay special at-tention to the social worker's role in nonclinical settings such as child-care centers and school-based mental health programs.

In Chapter 8 we develop a perspective on clinical social work psy-chotherapy that is informed by the conceptual framework we have pre-sented. We include newly emerging knowledge about the brain's plasticity, which suggest that the attachment dynamics mobilized in the therapeutic relationship facilitate change at a biopsychosocial level. In this connection, we examine the neurobiology of affect dysregulation and offer general principles for assessment and intervention. We propose that effective so-cial work practice with adults and their families offers them new attach-ment experiences that enhance individuals' levels of neural network integration and, in turn, their capacity for affect regulation.

In Chapter 9 we provide three detailed case studies that exemplify the practice principles presented in Chapter 8: One case from child welfare emphasizing a psychodynamic approach; one from community mental health emphasizing a cognitive–behavioral approach; and one from a fam-ily service agency emphasizing a family therapy approach. In Chapter 10 we draw implications from our inquiry for social work education, includ-ing suggestions for ways to include this content in social work curricula. We argue that, in order for social work to educate clinicians who are equipped to meet the increasingly complex practice challenges of the 21st century, the profession must join other disciplines in coordinated ef-forts to integrate and apply newly emerging knowledge from wide-ranging fields toward the enhancement of human well-being.

Neurobiology for Clinical Social Work

Chapter 1

THE BRAIN

An Introductory Tutorial

IN ORDER TO BEGIN our exploration of the biopsychosocial matrix within which emotionally meaningful relationships develop, we start with biology and introduce basic concepts from brain science, or neuroscience, a topic largely neglected in schools of social work. We intend this chapter as a beginner's orientation and proceed from the assumption that most readers have not had extensive exposure to the various disciplines involved in studying the brain. By no means is this introduction comprehensive; rather we focus on those aspects of brain development, structure, and function most pertinent to understanding affect, its development, and its regulation. Those readers who wish to explore brain science in greater depth will find resources for further inquiry in the references cited in this chapter.

This is an exciting time to be studying the brain. The proliferation of new technologies has made it possible to explore the biological derivation of such intriguing mental phenomena as emotion, memory, and levels of consciousness. These tools bring researchers to a new frontier—an increasingly detailed and sophisticated understanding of how the brain is shaped in the context of interpersonal relationships, and, in turn, how the subjectively experienced phenomenon we call the mind arises from activity in the brain.

STUDYING THE BRAIN

Knowledge about the development, structure, and function of the brain has emerged from studies of animals, especially nonhuman primates, and from various methods of studying the human brain. Given their pertinence to understanding human emotion, affect, and affect regulation, we confine our review to the latter methods. This review draws primarily from the comprehensive methodological descriptions provided by Nelson and Bloom (1997).

The least invasive of modern neuroscientific methods is *neuropsychology*, which involves testing hypotheses based on inferences about which areas of the brain are related to particular behaviors. Experiments may be used to compare the performance of a nonclinical with a clinical population on a given cognitive task, or to compare the performance of an individual on a cognitive task under different conditions (e.g., "eyes open" vs. "eyes closed"). Because areas of the brain involved in specific tasks can only be inferred, such experiments can only indirectly relate brain structure and function and, therefore, are less precise than some other methods.

Researchers employing *electrophysiology* attempt to relate observed electrical brain activity to ongoing mentation or emotion by observing *when* neurological activity is occurring. The invasive form of this method involves direct electrical stimulation of parts of the brain and recording associated responses. Because of its invasiveness, this method is typically employed with animals or with people already exposed to the risks of neurosurgery. More widely used in human brain research are two noninvasive electrophysiological techniques, the electroencephalogram (EEG) and the event-related potential (ERP). In both, electrodes placed on the surface of the scalp record the brain's background electrical activity. The EEG records activity associated with phenomena that are not time-bound, such as the experience or expression of emotion. The ERP, in contrast, is useful in tracking electrical activity related to some discretely presented stimulus—for example, a brief flash of light—and has been used to study such phenomena as infant cognitive abilities.

Two recently developed techniques of *functional neuroimaging* provide "pictures" of the brain's functioning that vary in their level of resolution and specificity. In positron emission tomography (PET) scans, a small amount of a radioactive substance that acts as fuel for the brain (e.g., oxygen or glucose) is injected into a subject's bloodstream. Presumably the region performing a particular function will require more of the injected substance, and, as the substance decays, electrically charged particles will be emitted from the part of the brain in which the function occurred. This method thereby reveals *where* brain activity is occurring under specific conditions. The invasive nature of such research poses obvious ethical constraints that prevent large-scale studies. Functional magnetic resonance imaging (fMRI) does not require exposure to radiation and is entirely noninvasive—and therefore safer and more suitable for research on nonclinical as well as clinical samples. This technique is based on the observation that, when a specific part of the brain is called on to perform some task (e.g., respond to a visual stimulus), that part will receive increased blood flow and thereby increased oxygen. Multiple images produced by the MRI scanner reveal fluctuations in oxygen levels that help researchers pinpoint those brain regions most active in relation to the behavior under study.

In essence, electrophysiological and neuroimaging techniques provide assessments of the flow of various forms of energy throughout the brain. These tools for determining the degree and localization of brain arousal and activation give researchers access to information about the ways in which the brain creates the mental processes that shape our subjective experience of our lives and relationships (Siegel, 1999). Thanks to these technological advances, we know more than ever before about how the brain is structured and how it works.

THE STRUCTURE OF THE BRAIN

The technological sophistication of tools for studying the brain only underscores a general sense that it is formidably complicated and defies

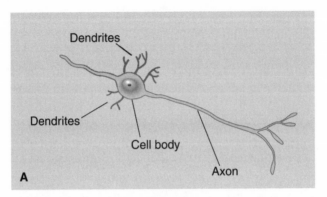

Figure 1.1   A diagram of a human neuron, the basic cell of the brain. The neuron is composed of a long axon, a cell body, and dendrites. Neurotransmitters are released from the dendrites, the branching ends of the neuron, into the space between neurons, called the synapse. Neurotransmitters travel through the synapse, then attach to an adjacent neuron's dendrites, which receive signals from adjacent neurons. Reuptake sites (where medications such as Prozac work) suck the neurotransmitters up into the neuron.

understanding. It is important, therefore, to demystify the brain. We begin with a reminder that, in most respects, the brain is an organ like the liver or the stomach and, like them, is composed of interconnected cells. Brain cells, or *neurons*, maintain an electrical charge and are composed of three parts: the *cell body*, which contain the substances that govern its metabolism; hundreds of branching appendages, called *dendrites*; and a single appendage called an *axon* (see Figure 1.1). Neurons connect to each other in the following manner: The axon of one neuron forms a link with a dendrite of another neuron; the axon of this neuron, in turn, connects with the dendrite of another, and so on. Because each dendrite on a cell body can accept multiple axon terminals, vast numbers of connections are possible (Pliszka, 2003; Solms & Turnbull, 2002). The brain is estimated to have 1 hundred billion neurons, each with up to 10,000 connections to other neurons, resulting in a potential matrix of *1 million billion* connections (Siegel, 1999).

Neural systems are constructed in the process of *synaptogenesis*, which works as follows: At the juncture where the axon of one neuron connects with the dendrite of another, there is a minute gap, or *synapse*, over which chemical molecules, called *neurotransmitters,* pass from one neuron to the next. The transmission of small amounts of neurotransmitter from one neuron to another is referred to as *firing*. Firing is the way neurons transmit energy and information to each other, and they do so constantly and simultaneously (Pally, 2000). Even when not receiving stimulation from each other, neurons fire at regular intervals in what is referred to as a base firing rate. But two types of neurotransmitter modify this base rate: excitatory types, which increase the chances that a neighboring neuron will fire; and inhibitory types, which reduce the chances of another neuron firing. Primary excitatory neurotransmitters include glutamate and aspartate. The primary inhibitory neurotransmitter is gamma-aminobutyric acid (GABA). Other neurotransmitters include dopamine, involved in motor action and the reward system; norepinephrine, involved in the fight-or-flight reponse and memory for stressful and traumatic events; and serotonin, related to the mediation of emotion and mood (Cozolino, 2002; Solms & Turnbull, 2002).

The neurotransmitter serotonin is probably the most familiar, because of the widespread use of antidepressant medications referred to as selective serotonin reuptake inhibitors (SSRIs). The way in which SSRIs work teaches us more about neuronal connection and communication. After a neuron excretes a quantity of neurotransmitter, via its axon, to another neuron's dendrite, the neurotransmitter is later taken back (think of vacuuming) into the first cell so that it can be reused. Neurophysiologists believe that it is the too rapid reuptake, or reabsorption, of serotonin that plays a role in mood dysphoria. SSRIs inhibit the reuptake of serotonin, keeping it active in the synaptic cleft for a longer period of time and thereby prolonging its effectiveness (see Figure 1.2; Solms & Turnbull, 2002).

This process of communication among brain cells just described is one of the features that distinguishes the brain from other organs. The other major distinguishing feature is that, although genetic programs play a large part in brain organization, it is interaction with the environment that determines the manner in which genetic potential unfolds (Siegel, 1999). As Solms and Turnbull put it, "The way our neurons connect up with each other depends on what *happens* to us. . . . The fine organization of the brain

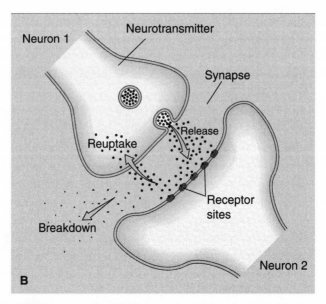

Figure 1.2 When a nerve impulse occurs in neuron 1, a neurotransmitter is discharged into the synapse (the gap between neuron 1 and neuron 2). This stimulates neuron 2 to fire when the neurotransmitter makes contact with the receptors on the membrane of neuron 2. The neurotransmitter is now sitting in the synapse and on the membrane of neuron 2. Neuron 2 will continue to fire until the neurotransmitter is inactivated. There are several ways that decreased availability might occur. One way is by reuptake, in which neuron 1 reabsorbs the neurotransmitter, thereby inactivating the neurotransmitter at the receptors. A second way is by breakdown, in which the neurotransmitter is broken down chemically and rendered inactive. In addition, there might be decreased synthesis of the neurotransmitter from its precursors.

is literally *sculpted* by the environment in which it finds itself" (2002, p. 11, italics in original). How does this sculpting happen?

Mental activities such as perception, emotion, memory, and cognition develop as circuits of interconnecting neurons become activated, or fire, at the same time and take shape as enduring neuronal networks. At birth, the brain is the infant's least differentiated organ (Siegel, 1999). As the neonatal brain is exposed to a new experience, be it external (e.g., hearing a sound, seeing a face) or internal (e.g., feeling an emotion, sensing a physiological change), new configurations of neurons become activated. Such experiences produce increased activation of synapses in *neural networks,* which, in turn, leads to the creation of new synaptic connections—a process called *synaptogenesis*.

Neural networks comprise one-half the volume of the *central nervous system*; the other half is composed of *glia*, cells whose apparent function is to facilitate the construction, organization, and maintenance of neural systems. The brain and spinal cord make up the central nervous system, and the autonomic and somatic neural systems comprise the *peripheral nervous system*. The role of the peripheral nervous system is to communicate between the central nervous system and the glands, sense organs, heart, and respiratory organs (Cozolino, 2002).

According to an axiom proposed by Donald Hebb (1949), those neurons that fire together tend to form the synaptic connections of neural networks, and those connections among neurons already weakly connected will become stronger. Infants are born with an overabundance of neurons, and a "use it or lose it" principle determines which ones will survive. Those connections forged and strengthened by repeated activation survive; those not reinforced die off as a result of parcellation, or "neural pruning." This process plays a major role in determining the manner in which the brain achieves its ultimate differentiation into various functional networks.

BASIC BRAIN ORGANIZATION

Before examining the brain's basic structures, it is important to understand its overall composition. The cell bodies of neurons tend to group together, and the resultant density of these cell groupings gives them a gray appearance (hence the term *gray matter*). The fibrous connections among gray tissues, formed principally by axons, are sheathed in white fatty tissue called *myelin* and comprise the brain's white matter. The cell bodies of gray matter group together either as nuclei or in layers. *Nuclei* assume the shape of ball-like clusters of cell bodies, whereas *layers* form when the cell bodies assemble in rows. The layers of cells typically appear on the outer surface of the brain (its cortex), and the folding of these layers gives the brain its distinctive wavy appearance. Nuclei lie beneath the layers of cortex, and the strings of white matter connect the two (Solms & Turnbull, 2002).

Mirroring its evolutionary history, the brain's structures have developed hierarchically from older to newer, lower (primitive) to higher (advanced), and their positioning in the skull reflects this evolution. At the base of the brain we find the *lower structures*, which include the neural circuits of the *brainstem*, a direct extension of the spinal cord. The brain's "oldest" structure in evolutionary terms, the brainstem is responsible for monitoring and regulating basic physiological processes such as heart rate, respiration, body temperature, and sleep cycles. Atop the brainstem is the *thalamus*, the reception center for incoming sensory information, which has an extensive network of connections to other parts of the brain (Siegel, 1999; Solms & Turnbull, 2002).

The "newest" and most advanced parts of the brain constitute the *higher structures*, principally the *cerebral cortex* found on the outer layer of the brain. This area of the brain is responsible for the formation of ideas and mental representations of self, others, and the environment; it is sculpted *postnatally*, in the context of positive and negative interactions with the social and physical environments. The cerebral cortex is made up of two large hemispheres that are connected by filaments of white matter, called the *corpus collosum*. Although the two hemispheres appear identical, they differ functionally. The right hemisphere specializes in processing global aspects of information: It gets the "big picture" of a situation, therefore rendering it particularly adept at processing emotional experience, expressions of nonverbal communication such as gesture or tone of voice, and somatic sensations such as touch, pressure, and overall body positioning. The left hemisphere, in contrast, specializes in identifying and processing the details of a situation and is therefore superior in processing the semantic aspects of language, making causal connections between phenomena, and coordinating fine motor movements (Pally, 2000; Siegel, 1998).

The cerebral cortex is divided into four lobes, each with different functions and each represented in both hemispheres (Figure 1.3). The four are (1) the *occipital* lobe, involved in processing visual stimuli; (2) the *temporal* lobe, which mediates auditory, language, and memory functions; (3) the *parietal* lobe, which links sensory and motor functions and

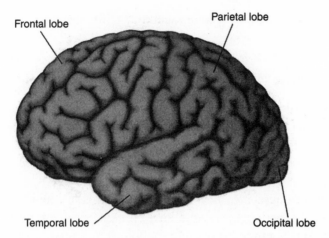

Frontal lobe Parietal lobe

Temporal lobe Occipital lobe

Figure 1.3   The four lobes of the cerebral cortex, as seen from the left side of the brain.

provides a sense of the spatial location of the body; and (4) the *frontal* lobe, sometimes called the "executive center" of the brain, which mediates motor behavior, language, abstract reasoning, and directed attention (Cozolino, 2002).

Lying between, and coordinating the activity of, the brainstem and the cerebral cortex is the *limbic system*. Key regions of this system include the *orbitofrontal cortex*, the *anterior cingulate*, and the *amygdala*. These regions perform the function of integrating and regulating a wide variety of mental and emotional processes, including attachment, and are believed to potentiate the human capacity for assigning meaning to internal and external stimuli. The limbic system is also home to the *hippocampus*, a subsystem that mediates access to conscious forms of memory (Siegel, 1999).

Of particular importance to affect regulation is the orbitofrontal cortex, located at the apex of the limbic system where the cortex and subcortical areas converge. *Orbital* refers to the position of this region, just behind the orbit of the eye. This part of the brain is believed to be crucial in such functions as social adjustment, the control of mood, registering affective responses to events, and storing them in implicit memory. It is expanded in the right hemisphere, dominant for unconscious processes, and contains neurons that process facial and vocal information. The orbitofronal cortex has been called the "senior executive" of the social–emotional brain (Schore, 2003b).

HOW THE BRAIN PROCESSES INFORMATION

The lower, central, and higher regions of the brain are richly interconnected via networks of neurons that form what Edelman referred to as reentry circuits (1989; as cited in Pally, 2000). These circuits relay information processed in specific brain regions to other regions in a bidirectional manner. In further describing the manner in which regions of the brain intercommunicate, Siegel (1999) noted that, as the brain receives stimuli from experience with the environment, signals from the brainstem that convey physiological information from the body are processed and integrated by the various areas of the limbic system. These areas, in turn, feed emotional and somatic input to the cerebral cortex, which also processes information from sensory, conceptual, and linguistic centers. The task here is to receive different neural "codes," coordinate the encoded information, and translate it into transformed neural activity that is communicated to the relevant brain regions as representations.

While processing incoming information generated by experience, the brain is simultaneously being *shaped* by the incoming information. Processed input "used" by the brain creates or strengthens synaptic interconnections, according to the "use it or lose it" principle described earlier. In this way the brain becomes increasingly differentiated. Siegel concluded that *"Experience can shape not only what information enters the mind, but the way in which the mind develops the ability to process that information"* (1999, p. 16, italics in original).

One example of this phenomenon that is particularly pertinent to the study of relationship development and dynamics is the information-processing role of the right orbitofrontal cortex. This area of the cortex is extensively interconnected with other limbic areas and acts as an "association cortex" for the limbic system (Schore, 1996, p. 67). Its circuitry is notably expanded in the right hemisphere and is believed to play a central role in the processing, behavioral expression, and regulation of emotional information. The right orbitofrontal cortex is involved in processing social signals and the pleasurable qualities of social interaction, including attachment interactions. It contains neurons that fire specifically in response to the emotional expressions of faces. By creating and strengthening synaptic connections, repeated face-to-face gaze, vocal, and smiling transactions between infant and caregiver directly influence the "hard wiring" of the infant's brain. Based on this model of neural network development, Schore concluded that the child's first relationship with the primary caregiver *"acts as a template for the imprinting of circuits in the child's emotion-processing right brain, thereby permanently shaping the individual's adaptive or maladaptive capacities to enter into all later emotional relationships"* (1997b, p. 30, italics in original).

THE COCONSTRUCTION OF THE SOCIAL BRAIN

At birth, the wiring of the brain is incomplete (Post, Weiss, Smith, & Li, 1997), and its progress toward organization is dependent, in large part, on relational experience. Research in neurobiology brings increasingly rigorous empirical methods to the study of the relational matrix for affect regulation and its correlates in brain development. This work reflects the view that the brain develops more rapidly postnatally than was previously believed, and that early caregiving experiences comprise the most salient environmental influence on processes of synaptogenesis (Schore, 1994; Zuckerman, 1997).

Early caregiving experiences affect synaptogenesis in three primary ways. First, during infancy and early childhood important interconnections are constructed between brain systems. For example, neuronal links are established between the cortex and the limbic system. The quality of a child's caregiving experiences may "charge" these neural circuits with either positive or negative affects. Second, whereas the absolute number of neurons does not change from birth to 3 years of age, the number of *connections* between these cells is predicated on a child's experience and the quality of stimulation he or she receives. The number of connections between cells reaches a peak at around 2–3 years of age and falls to about half that number by the time a child's brain matures to its adult form, from 14 to 15 years of age (Zuckerman, 1997).

Third, as noted, the child's developing brain operates on a "use it or lose it" principle (Galinsky, 1998), in that connections that are not activated through experience may be lost. That is, healthy early synaptogenesis is "experience-dependent" (Greenough & Black, 1992). Here, neuronal connections are generated and particularized, or adapted, to the repeated presentataion of particular and potentially idiosyncratic environmental characteristics. As Nelson and Bloom (1997) noted, the available neuronal cells at birth also form an expectant environment in which connections must be forged and confirmed in early life. So-called "experience-expectant" synaptogenesis (Greenough, & Black, 1992) occurs during minimal, non-particularized exposure to critical stimuli. An example is the way in which normative exposure to visual stimuli supports the development of depth perception. These types of synaptogenesis describe the two major mechanisms by which environmental input shapes the number and quality of neuronal links made during early brain development. The first 3 years of life constitute an overarching critical or "sensitive" period for these key processes. "Everyday caregiving" (Zuckerman, 1997), much like Winnicott's (1965c) "good-enough mothering," serves as the relational base and context for these processes.

SENSITIVE PERIODS IN BRAIN DEVELOPMENT

Within the sensitive 0-to-3-year parameter for brain development are different critical periods of growth and development for different regions of the brain. For example, in order for differentiated perceptual capacities to emerge, areas of the sensory cortex must receive specific types of stimulation (e.g., the visual cortex, in face-to-face infant–caregiver gaze interactions) within a specific time-frame (Pally, 2000). The apparent sensitive period for the development of the orbitofrontal cortex is between 6 months and 1 year, with a major maturational surge at 10–12 months (Schore, 1996). In order for the "wiring" of this area of the cortex to proceed normally, the infant must be engaged in exciting, intensely pleasurable, face-to-face interactions with a caregiver. Schore (1994) asserted that the resulting high states of arousal, modulated within tolerable limits by attuned affective responses by the caregiver, induce the growth of dopamine-releasing axons that grow from their cell bodies in the midbrain to regions of the orbitofrontal cortex. The increased amounts of dopamine stimulate increased synaptic connections among the neurons in this region.

It was assumed that the brain was unable to produce new neurons, a process referred to as *neurogenesis*, after birth. Environmental stimulation was thought to increase the number and strength of interconnections among neurons, but not their number, per se. However, research has revealed that in the hippocampus, the area of the limbic system involved in long-term memory, new neurons indeed do grow, even into adulthood, as the result of experiences with the environment (Pally, 2000). Nevertheless, it is clear that the interconnected systems of the brain undergo their most notable transformations in infancy and early childhood, as evidenced by the higher level of metabolism in the brains of infants than in those of adults. So although the brain is believed to retain a certain degree of plasticity throughout life, early childhood experience constitutes a sensitive period for brain organization and structure, because the brain is in its most rapidly evolving formative stages.

THE BRAIN AS A NONLINEAR DYNAMIC SYSTEM

Although our introduction to the brain is brief and elementary—a sketch more than a fleshed-out portrait—it nevertheless conveys the remarkable complexity involved in the brain's structure and function. As a whole, the brain functions as a dynamic system that is composed of subsystems. Neuroscientists have turned to nonlinear dynamic systems theory, also referred to as complexity or chaos theory, as the conceptual framework that best characterizes the brain's functioning (Schore, 1994, 1997b; Siegel, 1999). Complex systems function in a dynamic, constantly active, ever-changing manner and move in discontinuous steps from simplicity to increasing complexity. They are nonlinear, in that a small alteration in environmental input can lead to large and unpredictable alterations in output. They are open to, indeed require, interaction with the environment, can respond and adapt to environmental changes, and become linked functionally to other systems.

Complexity theory suggests that the brain is an open, nonlinear dynamic system whose adaptive development and self-organization depend on attuned interactions with caregivers. Neuroscientists believe that the intimate relationship born in such interactions literally promotes the development of neural circuits in the infant's brain. As Schore noted, "the self-organization of the developing brain occurs in the context of a relationship with another self, another brain" (1996, p. 60). This relationship, in turn, functions as a complex system, a conceptualization we explore further in Chapter 5. As a foundation for addressing these topics, we turn next to an exploration of the neurobiology of memory.

Chapter 2

THE NEUROBIOLOGY OF MEMORY

RECALL THAT IN THE Introduction we quoted Perlman's (1957) suggestion that relationship "leaps" from one person to another when emotion moves between them. Certainly the present emotional effect of one person upon another is part of this dynamic movement; but, as developed in Chapter 1, this present effect is colored and reshaped by each person's past experience of relationships — experience that, especially in infancy and early childhood, is likely to have become "hard wired" into enduring neural networks.

When a client first meets a social worker, his or her appraisal of the worker and response to the helping efforts extended will be dictated, in part, by previous relational experiences with those in helping roles. Especially salient, though outside conscious awareness, are memories of early interactions with caregivers. Although unconscious, these memories exert a powerful influence upon the way in which the relationship unfolds. If early experience has been positive, a trusting relationship may be easier to establish. If that experience has been negative, however, suspicion, wariness, and hesitation to become involved in the relationship may dominate the interaction and compromise the development of trust.

15

An understanding of the strength and persistence of these early mnemonic influences on present and future relational functioning requires exploration of the neurobiology of memory.

THE NEURAL TRACERY OF MEMORY

We all are aware of a variety of types of memory in day-to-day life. We remember a friend's telephone number, what happened at work yesterday, how to ride a bicycle, who our first grade teacher was, or how we felt attending the funeral of a loved one. But such recollection of factual information, skills, or reminiscences represents only the conscious level of memory. We are also deeply influenced and motivated by memories outside immediate awareness—a suggestion posited by Freud a century ago, which is now finding validation in numerous neuroscientific research findings. Whether conscious or unconscious, all these types of memory depend on the neural representation of information to which we have been exposed in the past, which can be activated for use in the present. Moreover, memory traces of previous experience influence how the brain will function in the future (Pally, 2000; Siegel, 1999).

These memory traces are laid down in the brain's massive assemblies of web-like neural networks that are capable of firing in numerous intricate patterns. These neural networks "learn" through an *encoding* process in which a specific set of firing patterns is activated and then distributed throughout the brain. If a certain neuronal firing pattern has been activated in the past, its probability of firing in the future is increased as synaptic connections among the neurons involved are strengthened. As Siegel concluded, *"The increased probability of firing a similar pattern is how the network 'remembers'"* (1999, p. 24, italics in original). In this way the memory has been placed in *storage*—that is, the probability that the same network pattern will be reactivated in the future has been increased. Memory *retrieval* occurs with the activation of this neural firing pattern that resembles, but is not identical to, the initial pattern activated in the past.

Siegel (1999) illustrated this encoding–storage–retrieval process with an imagined visit to the Eiffel Tower. On seeing the tower, the visual system of the visitor's brain responds with activation of its neural circuitry, thus creating, or encoding, a mental image or representation. Based on Hebb's (1949) axiom that neurons that fire together wire together, the synaptic connections forming this representation increase the probability that the firing of this neural circuitry will be reactivated in the future. The memory of the sight of the tower is thereby stored. Later, when recalling the tower, the neural network containing the stored image becomes reactivated, permitting the visitor to retrieve the image of the structure as well as other parts of the trip to Paris.

Siegel (1999) pointed out, however, that the contextual circumstances in which the image of the tower is recalled will alter the memory process. Rather than a literal reactivation of the past representation, the process of remembering will lead to the construction of a new neural network pattern. That is, the memory will be reconstructed in association with such variables as the visitor's emotional state and the present environment in which the recollection occurs. The resulting mnemonic neural network pattern will share features of the past representation, memories of other, perhaps similar, experiences, and influences of the visitor's present context and state of mind.

To the processes of memory encoding, storage, and retrieval, Solms and Turnbull (2002) added *consolidation*, a process that appears to be part of the encoding stage that continues into the storage stage. By consolidation, researchers mean that certain memories become entrenched at deeper and deeper levels of storage over time. This process may help explain why recent memories are most vulnerable to brain injury, whereas more remote memories endure postinjury. Consolidation also performs the function of sifting through the myriad perceptual stimuli we experience to exclude those deemed irrelevant. Many neuroscientists believe that much consolidation occurs during sleep, especially the rapid-eye-movement (REM) cycle of dreaming sleep.

SHORT- AND LONG-TERM MEMORY

The stage of memory storage is divided into several components according to the duration of time the memory is retained. *Iconic* or sensory memory, occurring when external stimuli activate sensory organs only long enough to lead to a perception, lasts less than a second. *Short-term* memory, also referred to as immediate or working memory, refers to information held only a few moments. The remembered facts or events may be present because the individual has just learned or experienced them, because they are being actively held in mind (e.g., holding an e-mail address in mind long enough to key it in), or because the person has consciously brought them to mind from longer-term memory. Short-term memory can hold a variety of pieces of information simultaneously and manipulate them as needed (thus the term "working" memory), an attribute that makes possible such higher cognitive functions as reasoning, decision making, and planning for the future (Pally, 2000).

The permanent storage of information constitutes *long-term* memory. In our example of the Eiffel Tower, the visitor's capacity to recall its image after the trip to Paris is over means that it has been stored in long-term memory. Pally pointed out that long-term storage "flows backwards" into short-term memory in order to perform tasks of searching for and retrieving information (2000, p. 48). Long-term memory is, however, "activity-dependent"—that is, if the neural circuits registering a memory fall into disuse, the neurons involved atrophy and die off through neural pruning. While this pruning process is particularly active during early childhood, it continues, to some extent, throughout life (Solms & Turnbull, 2002). If our Eiffel Tower visitor does not encounter circumstances that call the trip to mind, for example, over time, details of the experience may be forgotten.

EXPLICIT AND IMPLICIT MEMORY

Explicit memory, also called declarative memory, operates when a long-term memory circuit is activated and becomes conscious. It is accompanied by the subjective sense of remembering something. Explicit memory is divided into semantic memory (for factual information) and episodic or autobiographical memory (for recollection of oneself in specific episodes). By age 2, children can begin to talk about their semantic memories, a capacity made possible by the maturation of the medial temporal lobe, including the hippocampus, in the limbic system. The hippocampus is

especially involved in children's developing ability to remember the sequence of events and where they happened (Siegel, 1999).

Beginning at age 2 and progressing thereafter, children's capacity for
"mental time travel"—visualizing themselves in past, present, and future
episodes—becomes operational. This capacity evolves in conjunction with
maturation of the orbitofrontal cortex. The right orbitofrontal cortex, in
particular, mediates this type of memory, ascribes "meaning" to events, and
facilitates social cognition. Its development depends on attachment experiences with caregivers that evolve from contingent emotional communication (Siegel, 1998; for a detailed explication of the role of the various
brain regions in explicit memory, see Pliszka, 2003, pp. 92–103).

During the process of recollection, the hippocampal–orbitofrontal complex combines features of the time sequence, place, and subjective awareness of the remembered experience. This combining process means that
the resulting memory will not exactly replicate what happened in the past;
rather, it is reconstructed, and thereby altered, in present time. And the
more often we consciously recall a memory, the more "reconstructed" memory traces there are to be entered into storage, increasing the probability
that the initial memory will be further altered (Pally, 2000). This phenomenon helps explain how often-told family stories become elaborated or em-
bellished over time.

Unlike explicit memory, *implicit* or nondeclarative memory is "on line"
at birth. Advances in research on infancy make it apparent that, soon after
birth, infants perceive their environment, learn from it, and can recall it in
behavioral, perceptual, and emotional ways. For example, Schacter (1996)
reported research demonstrating that newborns will suck a non-nutritive
nipple more frequently when hearing their mother's voice than when hearing an unfamiliar voice, suggesting that they have retained in memory
sensory information about the mother's voice. Moreover, infants only a
few weeks old can transfer perceptual experience from one sensory modal-
ity to another. To illustrate, Stern (1985) described an experiment wherein
3-week-old infants were blindfolded and given two different pacifiers on
which to suck. The nipple of one pacifier was spherical in shape, whereas
the other nipple had nubs protruding from its surface. After giving the infants
time to gain some experience sucking one of the nipples, it was removed

and placed alongside the other. Once the blindfold was removed, the infants quickly looked at the nipple they had just sucked.

At these early ages, infants cannot consciously "recall" the perceptions leading to such habituation. The implicit form of memory does not involve the felt experience of "remembering" something. The effects of previous experience are present in the "here and now" but absent any sense of conscious memory. As Siegel noted, with implicit memory, "We act, feel, and imagine without recognition of the influence of past experience on our present reality" (1999, p. 29). Although nonconscious, the impact of this influence is profound.

The various types of implicit memory are mediated by different parts of the brain from those of explicit memory. Behavioral memory is activated by neural networks in the brain's motor cortex and basal ganglia, perceptual memory is represented in the perceptual cortices, and emotional memory relies on the amygdala and other limbic regions. All these brain regions are fairly well developed at birth and able to alter synaptic connections within their network circuitry in response to experience with the environment (Siegel, 1998). Only with later hippocampal development, during the second year of life, is explicit memory possible.

As noted in the examples of infant research reported above, implicit memory makes possible the development of mental models or schemas of experience that can be generalized across modalities (e.g., from feeling the experimental nipple with the mouth, to recognizing it visually). This form of memory also facilitates the capacity for anticipating what will happen in the future. An example of such schemas is the concept of internal working models of attachment proposed by Bowlby (1969). As described in the Introduction, these early-developing mental models, though not consciously "remembered," exert a powerful influence on the child's subsequent attachment relationships throughout life.

THE IMPACT OF STRESS AND TRAUMA ON MEMORY

Given that social workers encounter many people who have experienced acute or chronic stress and trauma, an understanding of the way in which these conditions influence memory is highly relevant to their practice.

Most clinical social workers encounter clients who have been subjected to highly stressful or traumatic situations yet seem oddly oblivious to their impact. They may report traumatic events without noticeable affect, or, though unable to recall the trauma, describe somatic symptoms suggestive of trauma-related aftereffects that linger as so-called body memories.

Different levels of stress and trauma appear to influence memory in different ways. Small amounts make a relatively neutral impact, whereas moderate amounts actually enhance memory. Excessive amounts, in contrast, can cause significant memory impairment (Siegel, 1998). Exposed to such stress, the body's physiological responses culminate in the release of steroid hormones, notably cortisol, from the adrenal glands. Research reveals that excessive chronic exposure to these "stress hormones" can damage neurons, especially those comprising the hippocampus, the brain region involved in explicit memory. Such prolonged exposure results in chronically elevated steroid hormones and leads to memory abnormalities reflective of hippocampal dysfunction (Schacter, 1996). Indeed, brain-imaging studies reveal that chronic exposure to stressful or traumatic circumstances reduces the volume of the hippocampus in people with posttraumatic stress disorder (Bremner & Narayan, 1998, as cited in Siegel, 1999).

As a result of such changes, people may not be able to recall a traumatic experience via explicit memory but retain the physical and emotional sensations accompanying it. Or the event itself may be remembered explicitly, but the implicit memories involved are disconnected from it.

Maria, age 23, and her fiancé, Bob, 24, sought help at a family agency for difficulties Maria was experiencing in their sexual relations. During the history-taking part of the interview, the social worker learned that Maria had been sedated and date-raped at a fraternity party during her junior year at college. She described this experience in matter-of-fact terms, displaying little affect as she recounted her story. She had no conscious memory of the rape; she surmised it after awakening unclothed on one of the fraternity house rooms. She went to the student health center, where she learned that, indeed, she had been sexually violated.

A brief period of counseling at the health center had been helpful, and Maria felt she had put this traumatic experience behind her. She

met Bob at the end of her senior year and became engaged the following fall. Despite Bob's gentle and patient approach to lovemaking,
Maria invariably became panicky and frightened when they moved toward intercourse. She experienced shortness of breath, heart palpitations, a sense of feeling suffocated, and was unable to proceed. In
individual work with Maria, the social worker's careful approach to
helping her give words to the affective body memories she experienced
during lovemaking gradually led to more satisfactory sexual relations
for the couple. By helping Maria make explicit through language the
implicit body memories of her trauma, the social worker fostered neural integration between the affective right-hemispheric networks and
those of the more cognitively biased left hemisphere.

As depicted in this example, dissociation between right- and left-
hemispheric neural networks is frequently seen in survivors of abuse and
other forms of trauma. Further, it appears that the impact of the trauma
is registered in the amygdala but bypasses the hippocampus, thus rendering explicit memory unavailable. In many cases, the implicit memory remains operational, producing impulses to flee, flashbacks of fragments of
the trauma, nightmares, or intrusive bodily sensations of the type described above; but autobiographical memory for the event is impaired.
This disconnection of aspects of memory can compromise future explicit
memory processing in ways that can, in turn, impair the capacity to learn.
Moreover, it can result in impairment of the process of cortical consolidation.

Although explicit memories of the traumatic event may not be stored in
long-term memory, the traumatized person may be subject to unbidden intrusive implicit memories, including flashbacks and nightmares. Siegel
(1999) reported research suggesting that nightmares may represent the
brain's futile efforts to consolidate the configurations of the dissociated
memory. Without consolidation, the trauma remains unresolved and the
survivor remains unable to narrate it in ways that could foster resolution.
Not all trauma revisits individuals in flashbacks, nightmares, or other forms
of implicit memory. Sometimes the trauma returns in the form of acting

out the unprocessed implicit memory, a phenomenon believed to be related to the intergenerational transmission of family violence.

Linda, a single mother of three children under the age of 6, was a participant in a community-based intervention program for high-risk parents and children. After being observed by the program's home visitor, Linda was referred to a parenting program in hopes that she could learn to adopt discipline strategies that did not rely primarily on the use of physical force. In talking with the parent educator, Linda was often heard to remark that she was "hit when she was young," that it "never bothered" her, and that "if it was okay for me, then it is okay for my kids."

In talking about her own childhood, Linda was able to describe experiences which the staff recognized as both physically and emotionally abusive, yet Linda described these memories in a very flat tone, without apparent awareness that such experiences are known to be associated with emotional distress and aftereffects. Because Linda's affective, implicit memory appeared dissociated from her cognitive, explicit memory of what these experiences were like for her, it was difficult for her to be empathic toward her own children's experience of receiving treatment similar to that she received during her own childhood.

A challenge for the social worker in this situation was to work toward building a strong alliance with Linda in hopes that, over time, she might be able to develop a more reflective stance about her own past that included the capacity to tolerate some degree of recognition and memory of the affective component of her own childhood trauma.

A major goal was to help Linda recall what it *felt* like to be a young child in her situation, so that she would not be driven to "remember" her affects through acting them out with her own children. It was as though Linda's affective memories were "trapped" in the amygdala and not available for neural processing by other brain structures, such as the hippocampal region. The worker's hypothesis was that the *implicit* memories of Linda's own early disciplinary experiences had been encoded neurologically. Through building a structured working alliance,

the treatment objective was to promote the neural network integration
of memories of her own experiences, thus increasing the salience of
the hippocampal process and *explicit* memory.

NARRATIVE AND MEMORY

In social work practice, clinicians typically invite clients to tell their stories, both past and present, in order to gather information for assessment
and intervention planning. For clients who have been exposed to extreme
stress and trauma, it is important to help them verbalize their symptoms so
that the clinician can begin to help link these up with the past traumatic
events. In this way, a narrative of the trauma is coconstructed so that its occurrence can be placed in a location and a time-frame. The purpose of
this process is to integrate neural networks of implicit memory with those
of explicit memory for the event. If successful, this integration makes it
more likely that subsequent implicit activations of the traumatic event can
be experienced as something that happened in the past rather than something that is inexplicably happening currently. This mnemonic synthesis
affords clients a sense of increased control over the symptomatic aftermath
of traumatic events.

The issue of "false memory" has become a hotly debated topic among
clinicians and neuroscientists alike. The controversy hinges on whether or
not childhood trauma can be forgotten and subsequently emerge in accurate memory some time in later development; or whether such "recovered
memories" are simply false, a product either of the person's creative imagination or of a suggestion "planted" by a clinician. The research reviewed in
this chapter suggests that trauma can impair memory processes in a number of ways, including the impairment of explicit memory for the event,
while the "felt" implicit symptoms remain. Pally (2000) suggested that a
present-day "retrieval cue" may trigger retrieval of "true" explicit aspects of
the traumatic memory.

Neuroscientists using different data assert that, indeed, recovered memories can be false. We know that children are suggestible, and some research suggests that false information about events can be implanted in
both child and adult subjects, then later recalled as a true memory

(Schacter, 1996). Further, depending on how it is conducted, psychotherapy can be a highly suggestive process. Excessive interest in, and persistent inquiry about, clients' traumatic experiences, for example, can put pressure on them to elaborate their stories of trauma in order to respond to the clinician's agenda. On the other hand, we know that many survivors of abuse have been silenced. Clinicians who deny or minimize the impact of extreme stress on mental functioning do their traumatized clients a disservice by failing to invite the details of each client's story. Such treatment can retraumatize clients, many of whom have been neither "heard" nor believed.

The false memory debate remains unresolved, but today's clinicians are better equipped to conduct effective assessments and interventions if they are aware of the issues in the debate and if they include in their case conceptualizations the various ways in which memory is experienced and expressed.

Having surveyed how neural memory traces are constructed, the different types of memory, the impact of stress and trauma on memory, and the role of narrative in memory construction, we turn now to a consideration of the neuropsychology of affects.

Chapter 3

AFFECT

Toward a Neuropsychological Integration

FOR OUR PURPOSES, we follow Moore and Fine (1990) in defining *affects* as complex psychophysiological states that are comprised of (1) subjective experiences of feeling, (2) cognitive phenomena, and (3) physiological manifestations. We think of *feelings* as subjectively experienced states, conscious or unconscious, and *emotions* as the outwardly observable expressions of these states. The subjective dimension of affects is typically experienced in feelings that have a pleasurable or unpleasurable quality. Cognitive phenomena generated by affects include thoughts, ideas, and fantasies. The physiological components of affects find expression in such autonomic nervous system responses as blushing, elevated pulse, sweating, and crying, and such voluntary nervous system manifestations as changes in facial expression, posture, or vocal tone and rhythm.

Given the increasing agreement among numerous disciplines that affect and its regulation are key to understanding the dynamics of human development and relationships, it is striking that this topic has been largely ignored in the social work literature. Regardless of the settings they inhabit, clinical social workers are dealing with clients' expressions of affect—anger, fear, sadness, joy, shame—in almost everything they do. Yet a review of eight textbooks typically used in social work courses in human behavior produced a reference to the term *affect* in only two (Berger, McBreen, & Rifkin, 1996; Newman & Newman, 2003). In each of these texts, the term was defined in one or two sentences but not elaborated beyond the definition.

This deemphasis of affect in social work scholarship may result, in part, from the move to so-called evidence-based or "empirical" practice over the last few decades (see Reid, 2001). Treatment methods emerging from this movement focus on observable and quantifiable indices of behavioral change, to the relative neglect of clients' subjective experiences and their affective expression. Moreover, in the current managed care context of practice, with its emphasis on brief treatment, many clinicians are required to conduct assessments and construct solution-focused intervention plans so rapidly that they have little time to attend to the slower-paced affective dimensions of relationship building. It is not that today's social workers do not recognize that dysregulated affect is a problem; what are often being ignored are the developmental processes by which the experience of affect and the capacity to regulate it are formed.

The need to trace these processes suggests important implications for history-taking. Only by understanding and inquiring about these processes can clinicians appreciate the difficulties their clients may have in making changes in terms other than "resistance." At the neurobiological level, for example, many of their strategies for regulating affect may be implicitly encoded and therefore outside conscious awareness. These strategies, although perhaps maladaptive, may have been mobilized to keep more threatening affects at bay. Attending to clients' relationship histories can help clinicians develop hypotheses about their likely affective sequelae in current functioning.

From an institutional perspective, the research we review here is also relevant for intervention planning and evaluation. Even when not fiscally required to conduct brief treatment, social workers are often in crisis situations characterized by the need to understand and engage complex, multiproblem situations in relatively short periods of time. This research suggests questions such as (1) why particular clients or client groups may find the relational demands of some interventions to be overwhelming; and (2) why the change process may not be linear. In terms of the latter question, people making progress toward change typically experience some affective discomfort and periodically regress in order to recalibrate their affect tolerance. Because the change process can be nonlinear, evaluation designs that look only for linear behavior change (e.g., from more to fewer compulsive rituals) may lead to findings that a given intervention was ineffective. Designs that include the clients' subjective experiences of the change process render the evaluation process more nuanced and comprehensive.

DEVELOPMENT OF AFFECT THEORY: CONTRIBUTIONS FROM PSYCHOLOGY

Although philosophers from Aristotle forward have made efforts to explore the role of basic affects in people's lives (for a brief review, see Fonagy et al., 2002, pp. 67–71), it was Charles Darwin who first turned the eye of science to affective expression. In *The Expression of the Emotions in Man and Animals* (1872/1965), he argued that various behavioral expressions of emotion had evolved in order to prepare the organism for action and, secondarily, as means of communication. Baring the teeth in primates, for example, prepares them to bite but also sends a threatening signal to an approaching animal (Demos & Kaplan, 1986). Darwin's findings about affect and facial expression went relatively unnoticed until the last half of the 20th century, when a handful of psychology researchers used them as a springboard for studying a series of basic affects and their facial expression in human beings.

Beginning with two volumes titled *Affect, Imagery, Consciousness*, Tomkins (1962, 1963) elaborated upon Darwin's work to argue that affects serve a primary motivational function. He was the first researcher to study affects in their own right, as distinct from cognition, memory, and other psychological functions. Tomkins viewed affects as somatically based, involuntary, automatic, and present from birth. He believed that they become psychological phenomena only with the infant's later-developing capacities for symbolization, reflection, and reasoning. Tomkins proposed eight "innate affects" that are accompanied by distinctive facial expressions and other bodily responses.

Positive affects, listed in their moderate and intense forms, include interest–excitement and enjoyment–joy. He regarded the surprise-startle response as a "channel-clearing" or "resetting" affect—that is, its effect is to interrupt the individual's attention to one stimulus and reorient it rapidly to another. The *negative affects* are distress–anguish, fear–terror, shame–humiliation, contempt–disgust, and anger–rage. Predicting contemporary research on the neurobiology of affect, Tomkins hypothesized that these eight affects are triggered by information entering the brain through its neural pathways, and that the density of neural firing—the number of firings per unit of time—is responsible for activating them. For example, he hypothesized that any stimulus with a sudden onset and a steep increase in neural firing will activate the startle response; if the neural firing rate decreases, fear will be activated; and if still less rapidly, interest will be activated.

Tomkins specified the facial expressions associated with each of the eight innate affects. The facial patterns accompanying enjoyment–joy, for example, consist of a smile with lips widened up and out. In surprise–startle, the eyebrows move up and the eyes blink. Distress–anguish is revealed in arched eyebrows, downturned mouth, tears, and rhythmic sobbing. In 1964 Tomkins published research in which untrained adult subjects were shown photographs of posed facial expressions and asked to judge which of nine affect categories (the eight innate affects plus a neutral, or emotionless, one) each represented. Correlation coefficients ranged from .631 for surprise to .988 for enjoyment, with an average for all nine categories of .858. The number of correct judgments made about each photograph reached statistical significance, and the robust overall correlation revealed a high level of consensus among judges.

A decade after Tomkins first published his work, his collaborators Ekman (1972) and Izard (1971) reported additional research designed to study the degree of correlation between the innate affects and specific patterns of facial expression. Later, Ekman and Friesen (1975) developed an extensive photographic atlas of adult facial expressions as well as a Facial Action Coding System (1978) designed to detect subtleties not readily apparent to visual perception alone. They reduced the number of affects in their research to six—happiness, sadness, anger, fear, disgust, and surprise—because their observations did not support inclusion of all of Tompkins's categories. In cross-cultural studies, for example, they did not find sufficient evidence to support his assertion that the affect of excitement is universal.

Slightly altering Tomkins's schema of affects by creating categories for disgust–revulsion and contempt–scorn, Izard (1971) found a high degree of cross-cultural agreement among judges matching facial expressions with presumed affects across American, European, Asian, and African subjects. There appears to a universal basis for the expression of discreet affects as well as their recognition by others—a conclusion supported by research in preliterate as well as literature cultures. Izard concluded that "the work of the present author and that of Ekman taken together appear to give clear proof of the innateness and universality of at least certain of the fundamental emotions" (1971, p. 266).

It is notable that the work of Tomkins and those researchers who followed him has not been more fully integrated into social work theory, education, and practice. The relative neglect of this work can be attributed partly to its relegation to academic psychological research. We suggest that this work is critical to practice because it can enhance the clinical social worker's capacity to make sense of and organize large amounts of nonverbal data. For example, knowledge of the affective correlates of facial expressions can help clinicians recognize feeling states in clients that they may not be able to express verbally.

CONTRIBUTIONS FROM AFFECTIVE NEUROSCIENCE

The advent of increasingly sophisticated technology for studying the brain has led to new ways of conceptualizing the categorical affects. Panksepp (1998), for example, designated four "basic emotion command systems" as hard-wired into the brain phylogenetically. The *seeking* or *reward system* is associated with the positive affects of curiosity, interest, and expectancy. This system activates curiosity in the external environment and generates the sense that something "good" will result from environmental exploration or interaction with others. It relies heavily on the memory systems that provide representations of objects and previous interactions with them, thus making it possible for the individual to learn from interactive experience. The *lust* subsystem is associated with the gratification or consummation of appetites (e.g., sexual arousal, hunger) activated by the seeking system.

The *rage command system* is activated by frustration of goal-directed actions and is accompanied by the negative feeling state of "anger–rage." It is expressed behaviorally in the fight aspect of the well-known "fight or flight" response and typically involves a facial grimace with a baring of teeth, aggressive utterances, a bold stance, and extended fists. Internally, there is increased heart rate and a redirection of the blood supply to the musculature, in preparation for violent action. When activated at a low level, this system may be expressed in a feeling of irritability.

The *fear command system*, centered in nuclei of the amygdala, generates feelings of fear and anxiety and is expressed in the flight response or "freezing" (in instances of milder stimulation). As in the rage system, these responses are accompanied by increased heart rate, shallow, rapid breathing, and redistribution of blood to skeletal muscles.

The fourth of Panksepp's (1998) emotion command systems is the *panic* or separation–distress system, associated with panic and anxiety as well as with feelings of loss and sorrow. This system appears to be connected with interpersonal bonding and parenting. The brain sites involved in these affects are believed to play a regulatory role in sexual and maternal behaviors in lower mammals. In animal studies, stimulation of the panic system produces "distress vocalizations" or "separation calls" and induces seeking behaviors. The bonding and parenting behaviors related to this system are governed by *social emotions* and constitute its *care* subsystem.

In addition to the care subsystem, Panksepp (1998) proposed a *play* subsystem, noting that children, indeed all young mammals, seem to require a certain amount of play. Play, especially rough-and-tumble play with others, appears to operate according to homeostatic principles similar to those that regulate sleep and other basic functions. Increasingly, play is believed to serve a crucial role in healthy development. Other social emotions, generated primarily in interactions with others, include jealousy, embarrassment, guilt, and pride (Damasio, 1999).

The Case of Fear

Thanks to groundbreaking research and scholarship by LeDoux (1996), the fear command system is the best understood of the emotion command systems. LeDoux studied experimentally conditioned fear in rats, believing that the neural structures, hormones, and autonomic nervous system reactions are similar across animal species. LeDoux's work revealed that the orienting fear-evoking stimulus reaches the amygdala in two ways: It first enters the thalamus and reaches the amygdala via direct neural pathways, a route referred to by LeDoux as the "low road." This transmission prompts the individual to begin to respond to the dangerous stimulus before fully realizing what it is or assigning meaning to it. Meanwhile, the thalamus also transmits information to the sensory cortex (the "high road"), so that a more detailed and accurate representation of the stimulus is created. The shorter thalamus–amygdala pathways allow the individual to react quickly to avert immediate danger, whereas the longer-acting thalamic–cortical–amygdala pathways allow the individual to fill in the details by applying cognitive processes of remembering past experiences with similar stimuli and making judgments about the extent of danger.

LeDoux (1996) used the example of an individual coming upon a poisonous snake in the woods to illustrate. Initially, the thalamus passes an indistinct visual image directly to the amygdala (could be a snake, could be a curved stick), prompting the person to take action quickly to avert danger. At the same time, a visual signal is sent through the visual cortex, allowing it to create a more detailed representation of the snake before it reaches the amygdala. In this instance, the automatic fearful response to the quicker-acting thalamus–amygdala pathways can avert a dangerous encounter.

LeDoux's discovery suggests that the neural pathways activated by a fear-arousing situation can bypass the animal's sensory cortex but still evoke all the physiological reactions to fear, such as freezing or elevated blood pressure. Applied to humans, this finding offers a neuroanatomical explanation for the phenomenon of an individual becoming afraid without conscious-ness of what has caused this affect (Gottlieb, 2003). LeDoux's formulation of a subcortical "low road" "suggests that emotional responses can occur without the involvement of the higher processing systems of the brain, systems believed to be involved in thinking, reason, and consciousness" (1996, p. 161). This suggestion has obvious implications for clinical work with people who present with anxiety disorders. Traumatized clients, for example, may respond with an acute fear response to stimuli associated with unprocessed implicit memories of earlier trauma (e.g., certain events, sounds, smells, objects) in the absence of danger in the current situation. In the following example, posttraumatic reactions were elicited by a major transition in the family life cycle.

> Richard, a successful 58-year-old trial attorney, came for help when, inexplicably, he began to have bouts of acute anxiety, vivid nightmares, and flashbacks related to his experiences in Vietnam as an 18-year-old draftee. He had clear memories of combat and recalled having similar symptoms for a few months after his discharge from the service; but he believed he had escaped the kind of lasting posttraumatic reactions many of his buddies described. Always an upbeat and focused person, Richard had returned from duty, immediately gone to college, and from there to law school. He believed in putting difficult things behind him and moving on with life. Following law school, he married and had two children.
>
> Richard's symptoms reappeared a month before his initial consulta-tion. Exploration of his current situation revealed that his combat night-mares and flashbacks began when his eldest son, 18, moved to a distant state to attend college. Consciously thrilled about his son's ad-mission to a prestigious school, he was at first puzzled by the social worker's questions about what this accomplishment meant to him. As they talked, however, it became clear that Richard's son's departure for college aroused strong affects in Richard, related to his own departure from home to fight in the war. Though he retained explicit memories of his combat experiences, the implicit, affective memories remained unprocessed. Extensive and detailed review of the emotional impact of

his experiences led to powerful abreactions of affect that eventually
provided symptom relief.

Affect and Rationality

Damasio (1994) has also advanced affective neuroscience toward greater
understanding of the intricate relationship between affect and cognition.
Based on research with brain-injured patients, he refuted conceptions of
mind–body dualism that imply a disconnection between affect and ra-
tionality. Specifically, he distinguished between innate primary emotions
and secondary emotions, the latter noted as generating mental representations acquired from experience.

Damasio (1994) suggested that the secondary emotions generate feelings, which he defined as mental images encoded in response to changes
in the body. He proposed that these bodily changes are represented as
images in the prefrontal cortices by what he termed "somatic markers."
Experience generates learned associations between external stimuli and
internal bodily changes, and the resulting somatic markers become part of
our embodied knowledge about how we feel. Subsequently, we may come
to associate a memory or thought with certain somatic markers, thereby
setting off the bodily reactions even though the original stimulus is absent.
A significant, emotionally charged memory, for example, can set off body
responses similar to those generated by the recalled event. Furthermore,
these processes can occur in an "as if" manner, absent external stimulation or conscious awareness. Such "gut-level" body responses, although
largely nonconscious, play a part in influencing choice-making, judgment, and other aspects of cognitive reasoning. From this perspective, previously proposed distinctions between bodily based affect and rational
thought disappear.

Indeed, Lazarus (1991) argued that affective experience cannot exist
without cognition, in that cognition causally precedes emotion in psychological events. He emphasized the role of cognitive appraisal in determining
emotional responses to events. According to this view, whether an individual experiences fear or sadness, for example, will depend on how he or
she cognitively appraises the stimuli triggering the affect. This assumption

about the connection between cognition and affect is the theoretical basis for cognitive–behavioral therapy. Therapists taking this approach believe that changing the way clients think about their situation can alter the way they feel about it. The assumption of a reciprocal connection between affect and cognition is also implicit in the research findings of some neuroscientists (Clore & Ortony, 2000; LeDoux, 2000; Zajonc, 1984).

Both Damasio (1999) and LeDoux (2002) have turned their attention to the affective neuroscience of the self. In *The Feeling of What Happens*, Damasio proposes three senses of self. The proto-self consists of nonconscious collections of neural patterns whose function is to represent the moment-to-moment state-of-body processes. The core self is based on core consciousness, a type of consciousness that provides us with a transient sense of self whose scope is events occurring in the here and now as they affect the state of the proto-self. For example, the brain of a person hearing a passage of music forms images of the melody that affect the neural networks of the proto-self. Core consciousness occurs when another level of brain structure generates a nonverbal representation of processes taking place in regions of the brain activated by the auditory stimulus of hearing the music. This representation enables a sense of knowing; the person has the experience of "this is me, hearing this music right now." The autobiographical self is based on autobiographical memory and depends on what Damasio called *extended consciousness*, a state of awareness that affords individuals a sense of themselves as continuous through the past, present, and future. In our example of the person hearing a passage of music, extended consciousness makes it possible to commit the moment the melody was heard to explicit memory and to anticipate that he or she might hear it in the future. Hearing the music becomes an episode in the person's story that constitutes an element of his or her autobiographical self.

LeDoux's *Synaptic Self* explored the role of synaptic organization in the configuration of the self. Noting that the brain evolves on the basis of the human genome as well as life experience, he subtitled his book *How Our Brains Make Us Who We Are*. The centerpoint of this theory is the bold assertion that the self is constructed through "synaptic processes that allow cooperative interactions to take place between the various brain systems that are involved in particular states and experiences, and for these interactions to be linked over time" (2002, p. 32).

Although providing rich descriptions of basic affects, their behavioral expression, and how they shape our sense of self, perspectives from psychology and neuroscience have not comprehensively addressed the development and subjective experience of affects. The most thorough elaboration of the subjective aspect of affects is found in insights from psychoanalysis and psychoanalytically informed developmental theory.

CONTRIBUTIONS FROM PSYCHOANALYSIS

In the late 19th century Freud began to write about affect from a psychoanalytic perspective. In early work (1893/1966, 1905/1953) he conceptualized affect as a quantity of energy related to psychic phenomena. The primary function of the psychic apparatus was to minimize excessive excitations. In this formulation, Freud cast affects in the role of discharging psychic energy associated with the drives. In 1917 Freud introduced a subjective dimension to his ideas about affect: "An affect includes in the first place particular motor innervations or discharges and secondly certain feelings; the latter are of two kinds—perceptions of the motor actions that have occurred and the direct feelings of pleasure and unpleasure which, as we say, give the affect its keynote" (1963, p. 395). In 1924 he suggested that the subjective experience of affect might be associated with the rhythms, sequences, rises and falls, and other changes in the quantity of the stimulus.

In *Inhibitions, Symptoms, and Anxiety*, Freud (1926/1959) introduced his second major concept of the function of affects: He identified their signaling function, suggesting specifically that anxiety could serve as a signal to the ego to mobilize its modulating functions and defenses. In this paper, prescient of LeDoux's (1996) work, he also emphasized the adaptive cognitive dimension of affect, hypothesizing that the idea of danger, for example, could evoke the affect of anxiety as a signal to activate defensive or escape behaviors.

Summing up Freud's two major streams of thought about affect, Fonagy et al. (2002) noted that in the first conceptualization he viewed affects as powerful, instinctually based, and dangerous forces that eluded conscious control. In the second conceptualization, in contrast, he saw affects as signals whose strength could be regulated by the ego.

These contributions notwithstanding, Freud recognized that his theory of affects was incomplete and left many issues unresolved. In 1936 Anna Freud (1946) extended her father's second conceptualization by proposing that the modulation of affect is one of the ego's key adaptive functions. Among post-Freudians writing about affects in the 1970s, Brenner (1974) offered a formulation representing a combination of cognitive theory and drive theory. He portrayed affects as evolving from internally generated instinctual processes of drive tension and discharge that, with development, become associated cognitively with memories and ideas. More recent psychoanalytic scholarship on affects has emphasized its adaptive functions (Emde, 1980). Nevertheless, Demos and Kaplan concluded that "psychoanalytic theories of affect have suffered from their inability to encompass the full range of normal, nonpathological affect experience and dynamics" (1986, p. 159).

The emphasis on a pathology-oriented, nonadaptive view of affects derives from what has been called the one-person psychology of classical psychoanalytic theory—a theory based on a conception of the human mind as a closed, intrapsychic system of instinctual drive energies and their deployment among the psychic structures of id, ego, and superego. A greater focus on the adaptive role of affects has been facilitated by the epistemological move from this one-person model to the so-called two-person psychology of relational psychoanalytic theory (Aron, 1996; Greenberg & Mitchell, 1983). Relational perspectives on affects and their development can be traced to object relations theory, notably the work of Winnicott (1965d, 1975), and to Kohut's (1971, 1977) self psychology. Both these theorists were keenly interested in the dynamics of the affective bond evolving from the earliest infant–caregiver relationship. Though he did not directly address the role of affect in the formation of attachments, Bowlby's (1969) attachment theory is the basis for much of the contemporary inquiry into affect regulation and its neurobiology (Fonagy et al., 2002; Schore, 2000, 2001).

Interestingly, although never fully realized, a neurological conception of affect and its regulation first appeared in Freud's early work. In *The*

Project for a Scientific Psychology, written in 1895 but left unpublished until after his death (1966), Freud began to apply his extensive experience as a neurologist to the study of affect and motivation. Here he first proposed that affect results from the discharge of instinctual excitation; and he alluded to affect regulation by suggesting that such excitation, both internally arising and externally generated, might be regulated by neurological processes (Schore, 1997a). Though Freud abandoned his *Project* to concentrate on developing his revolutionary psychology of mental life, he remained convinced that "all our provisional ideas in psychology will presumably some day be based on organic substructure" (1914/ 1953, p. 78).

Psychological and neuroscientific research reviewed in this chapter appears to validate Freud's early conviction and brings the study of affect full circle to its neuropsychological beginnings. Although some contemporary psychoanalytic scholars express a concern that today's focus on the neurobiology of mental life will rob psychoanalytic theory of its soul (e.g., see Frattaroli, 2001), others believe that each discipline has much to offer the other by working toward cross-disciplinary integration. Schore (1997a), a proponent of the latter view, calls for a "rapprochement" between students of the brain and the mind. We believe that such collaborative inquiry neither robs psychological theory of its soul nor reduces the rich complexity of human mental life to an artifact of biological determinism.

Nowhere has this collaboration flourished as fruitfully as in the explosion of multidisciplinary theory and research on affect regulation. Scholarship integrating formulations from object relations theory, self psychology, attachment theory, and neurobiology is illuminating the processes through which we come to know our feelings and learn to regulate them in relationship to others.

Only in the last two decades has this scholarship found its way into the social work profession. Object relations, self psychology, and attachment formulations have directed social workers' attention to affect regulation as a cross-cutting concept that can aid in assessment and intervention, regardless of the type of problem, population, or practice setting. Research based on these formulations demonstrates that even newborns are social beings; that they bring constitutional and temperamental predispositions that will shape how their caregivers respond to them; that caregivers' own attachment histories will influence their caregiving capacities; and that the nature of our clients' early object relationships and attachments will find expressions in the clinical encounter. Clients who have experienced relatively secure attachments, for example, will likely find it easier to trust the clinician, whereas those with insecure attachment histories may find it difficult to warm up to, and trust, him or her. Understanding that a client's difficulties in forming a trusting attachment may be encoded neurobiologically helps the clinician practice patience and focus on attachment opportunities with a "new" object as central to therapeutic success.

Finally, findings emerging from work in the cognitive neurosciences appear to erase the dichotomy between affects and thoughts. It is now clear that our thoughts are accompanied by corresponding affects, and vice versa. These findings have been particularly important in the support they provide to cognitive–behavioral approaches: They suggest that helping clients think differently about themselves and their problems can alter how they feel—and that such changes may be reflected in enhanced integration of cognitive and affective neural networks.

This multidisciplinary inquiry coheres around a fundamental assumption that how we feel, think, and relate to others across the life course is rooted in the ways in which we first learn to regulate affect. There is consensus that this regulatory capacity derives from the relational matrix of earliest infant–caregiver interactions and serves as the essential precursor to attachment. It is to the regulatory dynamics of these earliest interactions that we turn in Chapter 4.

Chapter 4

EARLY AFFECT REGULATION

Prelude to Attachment

THE UPSURGE OF ANGER, the flood of sadness, the mortification of shame, the rush of excitement—how do we control the intensity of these and other powerful affects in everyday life? How do children attain the capacity to self-soothe, modulate states of emotional arousal, respond adaptively to over- or understimulation by their caregivers, and, ultimately, manage impulses associated with aggression and sexuality? These questions are of central concern for clinical social workers, whose clients' difficulties with managing affects can result in problems ranging from domestic violence to substance abuse to mood disorders and other mental health vulnerabilities. The key to answering these questions is found in the concept of *regulation*, a theoretical construct employed by researchers in a wide range of basic and clinical sciences.

Learning to regulate the affects described in the previous chapter is a pivotal task of child development. Indeed, affect regulation—the attempt to maintain, moderate, diminish, or intensify affective states—has been termed "a central organizing principle of human development and motivation" (Schore, 2001, pp. 9–10). Gross underscored the centrality of affect regulation in human development by suggesting that "all be-havior is arguably affect regulatory in some broad sense" (1998, p. 287). Strategies for regulating affect exist along a continuum from the effortful, controlled regulation found in conscious coping mechanisms to the un-conscious, automatic regulation expressed in denial, projection, repres-sion, and other ego-driven mechanisms of defense.

As described in the previous chapter, many primary affects appear to be innate, and, as we explicate in this chapter, some rudimentary pro-cesses for the self-regulation of affects exist at birth; but the refinement and elaboration of these nascent inborn processes must be learned. This learning commences during the earliest interactions between infants and their caregivers. These early interactions, in turn, lay the psychobiologi-cal foundation for attachment, conceptualized by child development researchers as the dyadic regulation of affect (Schore, 2000). In nor-mally developing infants, attachment proper begins to achieve stability at around 7 months of age. This is the age at which the dynamic affective interactions between normally developing infants and attuned caregivers take the form of an intricately choreographed dance in which each part-ner follows the lead of the other in order to achieve a synchrony designed to minimize negative affects and maximize posititve ones. The steps of this dance are initially learned and practiced in the interactional precur-sors to attachment that begin with the infant's birth and caregivers' earli-est postnatal ministrations.

In this chapter we describe the affect-regulatory processes that evolve during the infant's first 6 months. First, we examine evidence of infants' inborn capacities for self-regulation. Then we turn to ways in which these genetically encoded capacities are further elaborated and fine-tuned dur-ing regulatory interactions with primary caregivers. We conceptualize these interactions as occurring within a framework of an interlocking infant–caregiver system, whose characteristics are best explained by the theory of nonlinear dynamic systems, also referred to as chaos or complexity theory. Throughout, we report research evidence suggesting that these earliest affect-regulatory infant–caregiver transactions play a major role in brain development by influencing the synaptic "wiring" of the infant's neural circuitry. With this theoretical integration, we attempt to demonstrate that, under normal circumstances, these early developmental processes set the stage for secure attachment, the biopsychosocial "anlage" for adaptive relationships throughout life.

EARLY PROCESSES OF SELF-REGULATION

There is accumulating evidence that the capacity for self-regulation is detectable before birth. Fetuses in utero exhibit various expressions of coordinated activity before the cerebral cortex is functional. Ultrasound films and observations of premature infants confirm that coordinated motor activity is evident in the second trimester of gestation and becomes elaborated in the third. As the fetal brain develops, neuronal pathways and chemical processes coalesce into an "intrinsic motive formation" (IMF) that, after birth, will organize the infant's consciousness and learning capacities (Trevarthen & Aitken, 1994).

Beebe and Lachmann (2002) reported research by Brazelton (1992) revealing that fetuses can change their state, lower their level of arousal, and put themselves to sleep in response to aversive stimuli; and, once the stimulation has been moderated, they can alter their state again—thereby demonstrating patterns of information processing. These authors also reported research by DeCasper and Spence (1986) demonstrating that neonates exposed to their mothers' voices during pregnancy can distinguish slight differences in rhythm, intonation, frequency variation, and phonetic components of speech at birth.

Self-regulatory functions of the fetus become more refined with the onset of the brain's "growth spurt" in the third trimester of pregnancy. Five-sixths of this critical period of rapid brain development occurs, however, postnatally, continuing for 18–24 months (Schore, 2001). After birth, the nascent self-regulatory processes apparent in utero become increasingly focused and complex in interactions with caregivers, and learning self- and affect regulation becomes a joint enterprise. As Winnicott observed, "There is no such thing as a baby" (1965b, p. 39), there is only a mother–baby interactional system.

The infant appears to be born with an inherent motivation toward contact with others, at first through smell, taste, touch, and hearing, and later through vision. Neonates purposefully and communicatively reproduce adult caregivers' facial expressions and motor behaviors, such as hand opening and closing. By making and breaking eye contact, they engage caregivers in regulating their autonomic state of arousal (Trevarthen & Aitken, 1994).

Beebe and Lachmann (2002) reported research demonstrating that, in the first 15 hours postpartum, infants exhibit information-processing devices that enable them to distinguish their mothers' voices (DeCasper & Fifer, 1980), smell (MacFarlane, 1975), and facial configurations (Field, Woodson, Greenberg, & Cohen, 1982) from those of other adults. Further, they can recognize their own vocalizations and discriminate between them and those of other neonates. In these rudimentary ways, newborns demonstrate an early capacity to distinguish themselves from others and begin to identify specific others with whom they prefer to interact.

At the neurobiological level, the newborn's brain is not only developing self-control and the beginnings of emotional regulation, but it appears to be predisposed to cooperative efforts that facilitate learning about the thoughts and feelings of primary caregivers. The neonatal brainstem, though apparently devoid of imagination and foresight, houses the basic motivational mechanisms necessary for engagement with others (Trevarthen & Aitken, 1994). These neurobiologial predispositions for interaction, in turn, further advance postnatal brain development. As Schore suggested, "the self-organization of the developing brain occurs in the context of a relationship with another self, another brain" (1996, p. 60). This process is orchestrated in moment-to-moment—indeed, second-to-second—communicative interactions between infants and their first caregivers. These first interactions, termed proto-conversations by Trevarthen and Aitken (1994), rapidly evolve toward the increasingly sophisticated mutual systemic transactions involved in dyadic affect regulation.

AFFECT REGULATION: A TWO-PERSON ENTERPRISE

Mothers appear to be primed to set the proto-conversations of earliest infancy into motion through their alertness to their infants' self-regulatory and communicative signals. At about 8 weeks, there is a rapid metabolic change in infants' primary visual cortex. This maturational brain change leads them to take an intense interest in the mother's face, especially her eyes (Schore, 2001). Responding to this heightened visual alertness, mothers seek eye contact with their infants and express joy, concern, puzzlement, and surprise in tandem with the rhythms of infants' changing affective displays. When expressing elation, the mothers' lively facial expressions trigger elevated levels of endorphins in the infants' developing brains (Schore, 1996). Mothers' speech takes on a breathy quality, with rising and falling pitch and intonation and pauses between utterances—a language described by various researchers as "intuitive motherese," "intuitive parentese," or "infant-directed speech" (Trevarthen & Aitken, 1994, p. 600).

Mothers are generally quite effective in discerning their infants' affective states, and infants begin to learn about the dispositional content of their emotions by observing maternal facial and vocal displays (Fonagy et al., 2002). These maternal displays also serve an affect-regulating function. Attuned mothers "read" their infants' affective states and attempt to modulate them toward a comfortable range through the medium of their facial and vocal responses. Simultaneously, infants, employing their own inborn capacities for purposeful interaction, are influencing their caregivers' affective states. The resulting caregiver–infant interactive system is comprised of three components: the caregiver as self-organizing and self-regulating; the infant with his or her self-organizing and self-regulating propensities; and the caregiver–infant interactive "field" with its own organization. The nature of this system is best described with concepts from nonlinear dynamic systems theory.

THE INTERACTIVE DYAD AS A
NONLINEAR DYNAMIC SYSTEM

Social workers have long considered the person-in-environment to be the primary focus of their professional attention. It is not surprising, therefore, that in the late 1960s and 1970s, they embraced general systems theory as a framework for understanding their clients' complex problems. General systems theory represented an attempt to capture the behavior of components of a system in mutual interaction (von Bertalanffy, 1968). This version of systems theory held sway in the field until the late 1970s, when social workers began to see it as too abstract for application in direct practice. Although criticism of the theory continued into the 1980s, social work employed its central tenets to develop more intervention-friendly models of practice adopted from studies of human ecology (Bronfenbrenner, 1979; Germain & Gitterman, 1980). Until the emergence of nonlinear dynamic systems theory, the resulting ecosystems perspective dominated the field as a framework for organizing data from the multiple systems of clients' lives.

Social work is now turning its attention to nonlinear dynamic systems theory as a more rigorously conceived and comprehensive epistemological perspective from which to view human behavior (Hudson, 2000). This shift in focus parallels one occurring in psychoanalytically informed infancy research and affective neuroscience. These disciplines are employing the theory of nonlinear dynamics as a biopsychosocial framework for understanding the systemic properties of the infant–caregiver dyad and, by inference, the client–clinician pair (Schore, 1994, 2003a; Siegel, 1999; Tyson, 2002). Capturing the manner in which the theory is being applied in the behavioral sciences, Schore asserted that "there is no dichotomy between the organism and the environmental context in which it develops. The physical and social context of the development is more than merely a supporting frame, it is an essential substratum of the assembling system" (1994, p. 63). This formulation provides an elegant and conceptually rigorous refinement of the person-in-environment perspective that has long characterized social work.

Nonlinear dynamic systems theory characterizes the way in which apparently chaotic disorder among parts of a system gradually becomes internally coherent and moves toward organization. As systems reach coherence and interact with other systems, they achieve new levels of integration that generate more differentiated systems. Resulting differentiated systems link together to comprise larger systems that, in continuing spirals of differentiation and integration, evolve toward greater complexity while retaining overall stability (Applegate, 2004).

Principles of this theory are particularly useful in understanding transitions from one stage of development to another. Such transitions are characterized by periods of instability, or chaos, occasioned by the shift from one stable state to another. A familiar example is adolescence, when various biopsychosocial stressors produce instability during the transition from childhood to adulthood. Emerging from a successful adolescence, young adults have achieved greater complexity in their capacity for adaptation and self-organization while retaining the basic continuity of their identity.

Self-organization, a nonlinear process wherein order and complexity create more order and complexity in a hierarchical manner, is based on the principal of primary activity. *Primary activity* refers to the propensity of living systems, although operating in an ostensibly chaotic manner during periods of transition, to achieve new levels of self-organization and self-regulation (Tyson, 2002). Neuroscientists now conceptualize the brain as a nonlinear dynamic system, and neuropsychoanalysts view the infant–caregiver dyad, as well as the therapeutic dyad, as a nonlinear dynamic system. As each partner in these interacting dyads affects the other's self-regulation, the inner organization of each achieves greater coherence and complexity.

This theory coheres around several key concepts. Those most pertinent to studying the biosocial aspects of the interactive dyad include concepts of nonlinearity, feedback, and sensitivity to initial conditions (Hudson, 2000). For example, when an infant first smiles at his or her caregiver, there is no direct cause-and-effect, or linear, relationship between the baby's smile and the caregiver's response. The caregiver is apt to do more than replicate the infant's smile: The smile is likely to elicit exclamations of joy and a returned smile that is affectively amplified into a broad grin of ecstatic delight. There is, in other words, a *nonlinear* or disproportionate relationship between the stimulus and the response. In turn, the caregiver's display is likely to amplify the infant's smiling response, perhaps producing a giggle as well. This sort of *feedback* process between infant and caregiver never settles into a regular linear, or negative feedback, pattern. It is never entirely symmetrical and is, thus, characterized by positive feedback processes. Subsequent infant smiles will likely generate similar, but never identical, responses from the caregiver.

In the interaction just described, the infant begins to learn to associate the smile with its internal correlate, a positive emotional state. At first, this association cannot be perceived consciously. But repeated interactions wherein the infant's positive affective displays are externally reflected in positive, affectively similar responses from caregivers lead to the infant's gradual sensitization to internal-state cues that match the affective expression. In other words, the caregiver is "teaching" the infant that smiling behavior is related to positive affects.

This teaching–learning process has been compared to biofeedback training procedures by Fonagy and associates (2002). For example, people have learned to control blood pressure, an internal physiological state to which they initially have no perceptual access, by watching fluctuations as they are mapped onto an observable stimulus. Repeated exposure to the externalized record of fluctuations gradually results in sensitization to, and possibly control over, them. Similarly, a caregiver's affect-reflective interactions with his or her infant provide a kind of natural social biofeedback training. Fonagy and associates (2002) suggested that this training evolves from a learning mechanism composed of contingency detection and contingency maximizing. Very young infants learn quickly to recognize contingency and behave in ways to achieve its maximum expression.

Infants appear to be extremely sensitive to contingent relationships between their behaviors and environmental responses. Fonagy and colleagues (2002) reported research by Watson (1972) demonstrating that 2-month-olds increased their rate of leg kicking when it produced movement in a mobile. Moreover, the experience of having control over the mobile's movement produced positive affects such as smiling and cooing. These authors also cited Watson's 1994 research demonstrating that after 3 months, the infant prefers less-than-perfect results from his or her actions. Apparently the novelty of slightly different results becomes more interesting than "perfect" cause–effect sequences. In the infant–caregiver system, this slightly imperfect contingency finds expression when the caregiver responds to the type and intensity of his or her infant's affect rather than providing an exact mirror reflection. Seeing her infant's smile, the mother might not smile herself but rather look surprised and exclaim,

"Oh! You're smiling!" The same *level* of affect is mirrored but not its exact replica.

Finally, the principle of *sensitivity to initial conditions* suggests that small stimuli, such as the infant's first smile, will likely generate larger systemic repercussions. The celebrating caregiver may call in other family members to witness this achievement, who, in turn, may phone or e-mail others about the exciting news, and so on.

CAREGIVER–INFANT MIRRORING

Although theorizing in advance of the development of nonlinear dynamic systems principles, the pediatrician-psychoanalyst D. W. Winnicott intuitively employed them in his evocative description of the manner in which caregivers introduce infants to their emotional lives through "mirroring" their affective displays. As he put it, "What does the baby see when he or she looks at the mother's face? I am suggesting that, ordinarily, what the baby sees is himself or herself. In other words the mother is looking at the baby and *what she looks like is related to what she sees there*" (Winnicott, 1971, p. 112, italics in original). Mirroring requires the caregiver to tune into the baby's internal world, "taking the disorganized processes within the child, organizing them for the child, and making them part of the dyadic interaction" (Cozolino, 2002, p. 196). In the complex systemic transactions of this early visual dialogue, the baby begins to learn the language of his or her own emotions.

Cozolino (2002), reviewing research by Jeannerod, Arbib, Rizzolatti, and Sakata (1995) that has identified "mirror neurons" in the frontal cortex of monkeys, suggested that similar neurons and associated pathways in humans may be involved in the facial, gestural, and postural mirroring proposed by Winnicott. Cozolino also reviewed research with primates reported by Perrett, Rolls, and Cann (1982), which demonstrated that a region of the temporal cortex contains "face neurons," or cells that become activated in response to faces and their expressions. Simultaneously, activation of neurons in the amygdala and orbitofrontal cortex contributes to the affective appraisal of mirroring interactions. Together, these recognition and affective appraisal processes help people (and other primates) distinguish friendly from unfriendly faces and the feelings associated with them. These findings lend support from neurobiology to Winnicott's psychologically based observations. As did Winnicott, these findings further suggest that mirroring interactions help us intuit the internal states of others in ways that potentiate the later-developing capacity for empathy.

The social feedback theory of Fonagy and associates (2002), described above, provides a useful refinement of Winnicott's original mirroring concept. They addressed the question of how it happens that the infant comes to interpret the caregiver's face as a reflection of his or her own emotional state. They pointed out that looking at another's face is very different from looking at one's reflection in a mirror. Indeed, as noted above, rather than offering a perfect mirror image of the infant's facial expression, the caregiver's visage will never perfectly match the emotional valence of what he or she sees, be it elation or distress. Rather, as suggested by the principle of initial conditions in complex systems theory, the caregiver will produce an exaggerated or "marked" version of what he or she sees—the sort of "as-if" or "not for real" display often seen in pretend play.

"Markedness" finds expression in the caregiver's "knowing looks, slightly tilted head, high pitch and slowed down, exaggerated intonation" (Fonagy et al., 2002, p. 296). These exaggerated communicative expressions act as clues to the infant, signaling that the expressions do not indicate how the caregiver really feels. Although exaggerated, the caregiver's affective response will be similar enough to his or her normal emotional expressions to enable the infant to recognize its dispositional intention. As Beebe and Lachmann suggested, this recognition depends not on perfect matching but on the infant's sense that he or she and the caregiver are *"moving in the same affective direction"* (2002, p. 95, italics in original).

When the temporal, spatial, and affect-arousal qualities of the mirroring social feedback mechanism move repeatedly in the same direction, the infant develops presymbolic schemas, or mental representations, of what to expect in subsequent interactions. In this framework, mental representations are defined as "more or less persistent, organized classifications of information about an expected interactive sequence" (Beebe & Lachmann, 2002, p. 148). In the infant's early months these representations are nonverbal and subject to the implicit mode of information pro-cessing. Rather than symbolic and verbally processed, implicit represen-tations are nonverbal, motoric, acoustic, visceral, and imagistic. Although presymbolic, they continue to influence how infants feel and powerfully shape their expectations for all subsequent interactions. In Stern's (1985) terms, they coalesce into representations of interactions that become generalized (RIGS).

The regulatory power of mirroring interactions is dramatically illustrated in instances wherein expectancies are violated. In research conducted by Tronick and associates (Tronick, Als, Adamson, Wise, & Brazelton, 1978), mothers and 3-month old infants were videotaped during 2 minutes of nat-uralistic, face-to-face play characteristic of their typical affective interac-tions. Following this period, the mothers were instructed to maintain an unsmiling still face and to stop vocalizing, thus violating the infants' expec-tations of contingent responsiveness. Initially, the infants smiled and cooed in efforts to reengage the mothers. When eliciting no response from the mothers, they typically turned away, almost as if they were trying to cope with the failed expectancy before making another attempt at engagement. After several such failed efforts to repair the disruption, the infants began to show signs of psychophysical dysregulation, often drooling, hiccupping, and beginning to cry. Finally, they appeared to give up, averting their gaze from mother, turning to the side and slumping.

When mothers resumed normal interactions after the still-face period, infants tended to look less at the mothers and maintained a negative mood, suggesting that the previous interactions had become internally represented (Tronick, 1989). By 6 months, infants displayed characteris-tic methods of coping with such failed expectancies. In normally occurring interactive sequences, there is what Beebe and Lachmann (2002) de-scribed as a reciprocal back and forth shifting between greater and lesser degrees of contingent responsiveness. When less contingent reactions occur, infants immediately try to repair them. This repair of disruptions in mirroring interactions tends to increase infants' feeling of effectiveness, adds to their repertoire of coping capacities, and contributes to a sense that they can remedy disruptions with other partners. These achievements help lay the groundwork for secure attachment.

Indeed, disruptions in interactive attunement and their repair constitute patterns of interaction that are essential to psychic organization (Beebe & Lachmann, 2002). Both in infancy and in later relationships, it is the rhythm of attunement, misattunement, and reattunement that constitutes the music of human relationships. Winnicott (1965c) seemed to be referring to this concept when he declared that mothers need only be *good enough*; were they perfect, development could not proceed because the infant would be deprived of opportunities to learn to regulate the emotions generated by failed expectancies. He believed that good-enough mothers (and by inference, good-enough clinicians) were required to fail in tolerable ways so that babies (and clients) could learn that failures are reparable.

Winnicott referred to maternal failures in adaptation as *impingements*. Minor impingements—the inevitable disruptions in normal, day-to-day interactions—are growth promoting and, as Cozolino (2002) suggested, potentiate neural development and integration. A flexible and expectable balance between gratifications and minor impingements becomes the psychological infrastructure for what Winnicott called the *holding environment*. Major impingements such as child neglect or abuse, on the other hand, overwhelm the child's capacity to integrate experience, compromise the development of adaptive coping strategies, and impair neural growth and integration.

It is important to recognize that impingements as well as attunements are expressions of the complex interactive caregiving system composed of two individuals. A failure to take into account the infant's role in shaping the dynamics of this system can lead to misplacing all the responsibility for impingements on the psychopathology of caregivers. An infant's temperament can predispose him or her to a lower threshold for negative or positive affect; indeed, some babies appear to be born with less adaptive regulatory capacities than others. Such differences can make it challenging for caregivers to strike an optimal balance in shaping their own affective responsiveness. In extreme cases, the baby with a disorder such as autism, which compromises his or her capacity to engage in reciprocal interactions, can generate reactive distress in the healthiest and most affectionate caregiver. In such instances, the caregiving system, rather than moving from chaos toward greater coherence and organization, may remain in recursive spirals of disorganized interaction, setting the stage for compromised attachment.

EFFECTS OF DYSREGULATION IN THE PRE-ATTACHMENT CAREGIVING SYSTEM

Even in less drastic situations than those in which significant infant or caregiver disturbances impair adaptive interactions, early dyadic dysregulation can get the caregiving dance off on the wrong foot in ways that have lasting effects. Fonagy and associates (2002) offered new insights on the origins of such dysregulation in pre-attachment interactive dynamics. Recall that, as caregivers mirror their infants' affective expressions, they "mark" their own responses through exaggeration so as to signal that what they are expressing is not how they "really" feel. Infants learn to distinguish these marked from realistic emotional displays and begin to develop categorically separate mental representations for each. They learn that caregivers' exaggerated behavior is only a representation of reality, rather than the actual reality, of their emotional state. This capacity to distinguish mental representations of reality from veridical external reality requires that infants become aware of the representational quality of internal states of mind.

At first, infants' awareness of mental states operates in an "equivalence" mode—what they are aware of inside is equated with what is going on outside, and vice versa. If caregivers respond to infants' internal states in an unmarked manner, infants may feel that their intense affects are contagious and universal. This manner of experiencing internal states can generate great distress because of the terror associated with the projection of fantasy onto the world outside. Unless this confusion of internal and external reality is overcome, the child remains in a mental state wherein inside and outside remain merged; frightening internal states and accompanying fantasies are perceived as "real" and dangerous. In the "pretend" mode, during which caregivers mark their mirrored affective display as "not for real," infants are helped to become aware that "feelings do not spill out into the world. The child's mental state is decoupled from physical reality" (Fonagy et al., 2002, p. 9). This decoupling makes internal states feel more manageable, thus fostering affect and self-regulation.

When, in contrast, the caregiver habitually responds to his or her infant's expression in an unmarked manner, representations of the pretend and equivalence modes remain undifferentiated. Due to her own unresolved conflicts, for example, a caregiver might react to her infant's expression of negative affect by reflecting the same affective tone, but in a nonpretend, realistic manner. The infant is likely to recognize the caregiver's response as his or her own actual emotional state. This failure of the reflective function will impair the infant's ability to form a secondary mental representation of his or her emotional state as not contagious. As a result, the baby will experience his or her negative affect as belonging to the caregiver rather than to him- or herself. Instead of helping regulate the infant's negative affect, the caregiver's negative expression will amplify it. Such amplification of negative affect in the infant will likely trigger another sequence of anxious, unmarked responses by the caregiver, thus further entraining dysregulated affect into the dynamics of the infant–caregiver system.

> Seventeen-year-old Monika had imagined that her infant daughter, Jennifer, would be cuddly, smiling, and adoring. But Jennifer was instead fussy, difficult to soothe, and reacted to Monika's touch by stiffening up and turning away from her. Monika interpreted this behavior as rejecting and angry and responded accordingly by yelling at Jennifer and forcefully holding her close to her body in efforts to get the baby to "melt" into her arms. Monika was not miming anger—she *was* angry. Jennifer seemed to intuit her mother's affect and became more agitated, cranky, and tried to push Monika away, thus further escalating her mother's distressed behavior.

In this case, the social worker might support Monika's sense of discouragement and empathize with her frustration at not feeling connected to her baby. Further, the worker might help Monika explore other patterns of interaction that might better suit the infant's temperament and interrupt the negative interaction cycle. For example, the baby might respond better to interactions that do not require her to be held so closely. Monika could be helped to follow Jennifer's lead in regulating the type and intensity of their play.

Fonagy and colleagues (2002) hypothesized that affect dysregulation also can result from interactions during which the caregiver mirrors back a marked but incongruent, distorted reflection of the infant's emotional state. This pattern can result from distortions in the caregiver's perceptions of the infant's behavior. For example, a caregiver might experience anxiety in response to the infant's excitement about physical contact and project a defensive emotional reaction, such as aggression, onto the infant. Having misinterpreted the infant's arousal due to her own defensive distortions, she might then respond with an exaggerated display of aggressive affect mirroring. One possible consequence is that the infant will connect the incorrectly categorized affect state expressed by the caregiver to his or her own emotional state. In this example, the infant's experience of positive arousal becomes associated with an aggressive display, putting him or her at risk for a distorted self-representation of his or her affective state.

> Thomas, a first-time father, had difficulty responding to his infant son's highly animated behavioral style. Nathan was a high-energy child with a vigorous physicality. When Thomas picked up Nathan, Nathan squealed, bicycled his legs, and flailed his arms. Rather than recognize his son's natural exuberance as an enthusiastic gesture toward connection, Thomas interpreted it as aggression and tended to become irritated. In these interactions he would display an angry face, hold Nathan tightly at arm's length, shaking him, and yell, "So you want to *fight*, do you!" After a few attempts to get his father to respond to his energetic approach and finding instead an increasingly angry face, Nathan would look tense, frightened, and bewildered; but soon his face assumed an angry expression. The social worker observing the pair became concerned that Nathan might begin to associate his gestures toward lively connection with angry feelings, thus mislabeling his inner state as congruent with his father's.

In beginning to address this obvious affective discontinuity between Thomas and Nathan, a social worker, equipped with knowledge derived from research on facial expressions and their affective correlates, might help Thomas notice his baby's bewildered expression just before displaying an angry face. Helping Thomas to tune into Nathan's bewilderment could increase his empathic understanding of other possible meanings of his son's behavior. The worker might reinterpret what is going on by saying, "I think he's really excited to be with you — it's his way of playing with you. He's not sure what's going on when you think he wants to fight, and it's that puzzlement that then makes him look angry."

Fonagy and associates (2002) speculated that chronic patterns of such distortions in mirroring may explain the developmental etiology of what Winnicott (1965b) termed the false self. In Winnicott's concept, when caregivers' own dysregulated affects impair their capacity to read the affective intentions of their infants' spontaneous gestures, they mirror back their own emotional state in ways that invalidate infants' experience. A possible outcome of such an impingement is that infants' "true" or spontaneous, creative self is hidden and protected behind a false-self facade. Having acquiesced to the caregivers' affective agenda, the infants may begin to experience their caregivers' gestures as though they are their own. The self presented to the world as a defense against anxiety aroused by this misattribution may be overly compliant. The compliant self may appear true, or real, but lacks vitality and originality. Children who grow up in this relational context often forfeit attention to their own needs to become caretakers of others' needs. As reinterpreted in the formulation of Fonagy and his associates, the development of a false-self defense in infants results from chronic interactions during which their awareness of their own affects is forfeited as they learn to mimic those of caregivers. This mimicry, born out of marked but distorted affect mirroring, may have a veneer of authenticity but is only a caricature of the baby's true self.

Beebe and Lachmann (2002) reported research by Beebe and Stern (1977) describing another type of early infant–caregiver misattunement that results from caregiver overstimulation and infant withdrawal. Four-month-old infants were observed with mothers who "loomed" into their babies' faces, prompting the infants to move their heads back and away. Responding to this mini-withdrawal, which the authors referred to as a "dodge," the mothers "chased" by moving their heads and bodies toward the babies. Their chasing behavior stimulated the babies to move their heads still further away. These interactions occurred in split-second sequences, in which the babies began to "dodge" even before the mothers had completed their "chase" approach. Bidirectional regulation remains present in this "chase and dodge" dance, but the *quality* of affective relatedness is compromised. As Beebe and Lachmann (2002) characterized this dance, the infant may want to stay close to mother but feels uncomfortably overstimulated when he or she moves in too closely. The mother, in turn, is likely to feel that her urge to connect with her infant is being rejected, leaving her anxious and disappointed and at risk of pulling away herself.

Recall that normal infants are born neurologically prewired to interact purposefully and communicatively with their caregivers (Trevarthen & Aitken, 1994). They initially seek affectively contingent contact through touch, hearing, olfaction, and vision (a little later). When they encounter the types of interactive dysynchrony just described without subsequent repair, their nascent sense of agency—the expectation that their own gestures produce affectively congruent responses—is truncated in ways that can compromise their ability to become aware of their own affective state and use that awareness to alter the state, if needed. In turn, difficulty discerning their own state will make it difficult to attune accurately to the inner states of others (Fonagy et al., 2002). Beebe and Lachmann (2002) suggested that expectancies of such dysregulation are stored in implicit procedural memory as presymbolic mental representations of self and other in interaction.

When clients bring such representations of self in interaction with others to the clinical encounter, clinicians must be prepared to "start where the client is" in terms of his or her unconscious expectations of relational misattunement. Given that the representations governing these expectations are presymbolic, the client is unlikely to be able to verbalize them; instead they will be acted out in the manner in which the client relates to the clinician—with suspicion, withdrawl, mistrust, wariness, or anger.

Because attachment is unlikely to happen quickly, the clinician must be patient and emphasize interventions that convey empathy for, and sensitivity to, the client's defensive, maladaptive efforts to regulate frightening affects. Such a clinical approach calls on the social worker to employ his or her own capacities to attune to the inner states of others.

In later chapters we provide detailed examples of ways in which social workers can employ clinical implications of this research in assessment and intervention, and we make recommendations for ways to incorporate scholarship about early affect regulation into social work education. First, having considered the precursors to attachment proper, we turn in Chapter 5 to a comprehensive review of attachment theory and research.

Chapter 5

ATTACHMENT

The Relational Base of Affect Regulation

IN TERMS OF THE EMOTIONAL life of the child, the emerging capacity for human relationships is a primary developmental task of the first years of life. As described in Chapter 4, the infant's capacity to engage in mutually regulatory relationships begins before birth and continues to develop in the context of early interpersonal experiences. The multidisciplinary study of attachment research has focused on the *quality* of these early relationships and their importance to the developmental well-being of the child. Although the nature of caregiving relationships changes as the child matures, the stability of the psychological tie between child and caregiver(s) is critical in ensuring the child's ongoing ability to master successive developmental challenges. Infants and young children who lack the opportunity for meaningful attachment relationships, or who experience disruption in primary caregiving relationships, are at risk for serious developmental difficulties. Thus, the field of attachment research is highly relevant to clinicians who work with many special groups of parents and children facing challenges to the formation of stable family bonds (Cassidy, 1994; Sroufe, Egeland, & Kreutzer, 1990).

58

The importance of early relational experience is being studied anew as methodological advances in the cognitive neurosciences have allowed researchers to examine the neurobiological correlates and consequences of early relational experience (Gunnar, 2000; Gunnar, 2001; Schore, 2000). Research describes the processes by which the repeated patterns of interaction that underlie the formation of attachment bonds are themselves associated with specific aspects of early brain development that shape the infant's capacity to *experience broad ranges of affect* and to *regulate states of psychophysiological arousal*. These capacities are core features of developmental well-being and important foci of the assessment and treatment of a range of emotional difficulties in childhood.

The purpose of this chapter is to consider the concept of attachment as an important organizational construct in the study of emotional development, its importance in the child's emerging capacity for affect regulation, as well as to demonstrate how this conceptual foundation relates to social work practice. Following a brief introduction, we review the major contributions of attachment theory to our understanding of the emotional world of young children. In particular, we examine (1) the origins of attachment theory; (2) Bowlby's attachment theory as a conceptual framework for practice and research; (3) individual differences in patterns of attachment; (4) developmental consequences of variation in attachment patterns; and (5) the intergenerational transmission of attachment patterns. Within this review, we focus on the attachment relationship as a mutual system of affect regulation.

The capacity for affect regulation is a core feature of infant mental health, and dysregulated affect is a core feature of many presenting problems observed by clinicians in multiple settings. Practitioners are likely familiar with the behavioral presentation of dysregulated affect in young children, such as that seen in temper tantrums, uncontrolled crying, difficulty in soothing and self-soothing, and problems with the delay of gratification and toleration of frustration. Moreover, as research in the affective neurosciences has demonstrated, early relational experience affects brain development in ways that shape the neurobiological substrate of affect regulation. Thus, studies on attachment and early brain development converge in their efforts to understand the processes by which the capacity for affect regulation emerges in the context of early interpersonal experience.

We also consider the clinical implications of attachment, including concepts of the internal working model, the nature of reflective functioning, and the importance of the caregiver's capacity to mentalize about the internal world of the child in ways that support the child's emergent capacity to regulate affect and approach developmental challenges with a sense of optimism and hope for the future.

OVERVIEW OF ATTACHMENT RESEARCH

The construct of attachment has been an important organizing framework in the study of child development. The advent of attachment research provided a conceptual framework for understanding the psychological importance, *to the child*, of access to stable and continuous caregiving relationships. An important element of attachment research is a focus on the developmental consequences of attachment, or the ways in which individual differences in the quality of attachment are associated with particular patterns of risk and resiliency in childhood and across the lifespan (Benoit & Parker, 1994). Many of the developmental outcomes associated with varying patterns of attachment are related to affect regulation. The capacity for affect regulation has long been understood as an important element of self-regulation and the capacity for adaptation in a range of circumstances.

A broad range of studies has long suggested that from the earliest weeks of life, infants learn to regulate powerful psychophysiological states in mirroring interactions with their primary caregivers. From different perspectives, theorists and clinicians have described the development of an emotional dialogue between caregiver(s) and infant that serves several important functions. Specifically, these studies have shown that when infants see their feelings registered and reciprocated in the facial expressions and behaviors of the caregiver, they learn to make meaning of and regulate their intensity. Thus, establishing the infant's capacity to regulate affect, or to modulate strong feeling states, is a key task of early caregiver–child interactions and a primary goal of early attachment relationships.

As we discuss in the sections to follow, even the earliest research on attachment construed primary attachment relationships as regulatory systems that helped the developing child to modulate psychophysiological states (Ainsworth et al., 1978; Bowlby, 1969). More recently, researchers have begun to focus on the processes by which differences in the quality of attachment are associated with patterns of risk and resiliency characterized by individual differences in the capacity to experience and modulate affective states of arousal (Schore, 1994; Siegel, 1999; Sroufe et al., 2003). One contribution from the field of attachment theory that is well represented in a range of clinical models is the concept of the internal working model. As we shall see in Chapters 5 and 6, many clinicians and researchers have utilized the concept of the internal working model of attachment to explore and address questions about the intergenerational transmission of attachment styles, and the ways in which early internalization of attachment models comes to light in the context of the therapeutic relationship. Specifically, problems in early experiences of attachment are sometimes represented in the therapeutic context in difficulties with engagement and trust.

The Origins of Attachment Theory: Recognizing The Internal World of The Child

The field of attachment research has changed our understanding of the psychological world of infants and young children and the ways in which early experience is associated with later developmental outcomes. The earliest studies of what is now termed *attachment* showed that both human and animal babies exhibit developmental disturbances if primary attachment relationships are disrupted (Freud & Burlingham, 1994; Harlow, 1958; Spitz & Wolf, 1946). Until the publication of these studies, the internal meaning, *to the child,* of the primary attachment figure was not clearly understood. These early studies laid the foundation for the interdisciplinary study of attachment relationships and the role of primary attachment figures in supporting the developmental well-being and psychological world of the child.

Clinicians working with children provided the earliest scholarly works that focused on describing the importance of primary caregiving relationships to the psychological and physical well-being of the developing child (Freud & Burlingham, 1944; Spitz Wolf, 1946). Spitz and Wolf (1946) described the psychological trauma and physical deterioration of children who were separated from their parents due to extended hospital stays. Anna Freud and Dorothy Burlingham (1944) described the despair they observed among children separated from parents during World War II, when children were sent to rural areas in an effort to protect them from war-related violence. Both of these reports described that functional caretaking that met the child's physical requirement for nutrition and warmth was necessary but not sufficient to ensure their well-being. Without the benefit of a stable relationship with a psychologically available caregiver, these children failed to thrive and showed a range of developmental problems. Specifically, these early studies suggested the importance of the attachment relationship to the child's ability to (1) tolerate psychophysiological states of arousal, (2) sustain investment in the external world, and (3) regulate affect in developmentally appropriate ways. As we examine later in this chapter, the "hidden regulators" (Gunnar, 2003; Gunnar et al., 2001) embedded within the attachment relationship are the focus of current psychodynamically informed work on the clinical implications of attachment, as well as of research on the neurobiological correlates of attachment (Fonagy, Gergely, Jurist, & Target, 2002; Schore, 1994; Siegel, 1999).

In summary, a history of research on attachment shows that understanding of this important mental and relational construct began to develop when clinicians observed the grief-stricken reactions of young children who were separated under difficult circumstances from their primary attachment figures. Early clinical research identified the importance, to the child, of affective bonds that are stable and continuous. Importantly, these early researchers showed that even when the children's physical needs were attended to, they displayed both psychological and physical reactions to the loss of important relational figures. Additionally, clinical research has demonstrated the important point that for young children, separation from caregivers constitutes a significant stressor, and that in the absence of a trusted caregiver, modulation of stress, anxiety, and other affective states is difficult for children to sustain.

Bowlby's Attachment Theory as A Conceptual Framework for Practice and Research

John Bowlby (1952, 1969) pioneered the field of attachment research with his ethological theory of attachment. This new theory was of particular importance because it focused on the affective, relational bond between caregiver and infant and the salience of this bond (i.e., attachment) for the infant's growth, development, and well-being. Bowlby's theory of attachment is considered to be *ethological* in nature because he believed that human infants are biologically predisposed to form stable and continuous attachment relationships with their primary caregivers. Bowlby observed that human infants, like many primate infants, required extended periods of parental care and support to ensure their physical survival and safe opportunities for exploration and mastery of the environment. Building on the infant's development in physical, cognitive, and social–emotional spheres, the attachment relationship extends the infant's pleasure in human interaction and provides increased opportunity for exploration and learning, as the baby learns to rely upon the caregiver's judgment and protection.

The field of attachment research has moved far beyond Bowlby's early description of the nature of the affective bond that forms between infants and their primary caregivers. Yet his work remains an important conceptual framework for many current issues in the study of attachment and human development. One aspect of Bowlby's work—his description of the child's *internal working model* of attachment (Bowlby, 1980)—has had particular relevance in moving the field of attachment research forward.

The construct of the internal working model refers to the developing child's mental representations of his or her early caregiving experiences. Specifically, the internal working model refers to the child's internal, implicit memories and mental representations of the degree to which he or she comes to expect sensitive, contingent, and warmly responsive care from primary attachment figures (Fonagy, 2002; Fonagy & Target, 1998). The internal working model has been a powerful concept in developmental work because it provides an explanatory structure for the ways in which early relational experiences may become internalized, carried forward, and represented cross-generationally. Thus the construct also reflects one of the most important themes in developmental psychology and developmental psychopathology. To clinicians working with children and families, the role of early experience in later development and the degree to which relational experiences are carried forward or are open to change is of primary clinical relevance. An understanding of the internal working model is useful in working with both children and adults. For example, if a parent develops a style of managing anxiety by turning away from important relational partners, he or she may be challenged by a child's need to turn toward him or her for aid in the modulation of the child's anxiety. In this case, it would be important to explore if the parent's internal working model of attachment impedes the use of relationships as an element of support in the management of affect.

As new research in the cognitive neurosciences explores the development and consequences of attachment, researchers identify the neurobiological substrates of the internal working model and the processes by which early interpersonal experiences shape memory, expectations about human relatedness, and the child's internal representation of attachment figures. This research reemphasizes the nature of the attachment relationship as a truly biopsychosocial system that is fluid and responsive to environmental and relational change (Greenoug & Black, 1992).

In summary, the work of John Bowlby has been of critical importance to the development of most empirical studies of attachment. As an ethologist, Bowlby described human infants as biologically predisposed to form affective bonds with their primary caregivers. Moreover, he detailed how attachment relationships fulfill the dual developmental goals of promoting physical survival and providing opportunities for both exploration and learning. Over time, researchers have demonstrated that children develop internal working models of their primary attachment relationships and that qualitative differences in attachment relationships are associated with a range of developmental outcomes that are critical to child well-being and development across time. This pattern of associations is being studied anew as we incorporate new research on early development and the role of relational experience in shaping developmental well-being.

Individual Differences in Patterns of Attachment

Bowlby conceptualized attachment relationships as organized to fulfill important developmental goals. The affective bond between infant and caregiver was understood to promote proximity between infant and caregiver and thus ensure the infant's safety and ability to utilize the caregiver as a secure base for exploring the world of objects and people. Building on the work of John Bowlby, other researchers conceptualized the attachment relationship as a mutually regulatory system that supports the infant's developing capacity to regulate internal psychophysiological states, attention, and affect. Sroufe (2000) described attachment as "the apex of dyadic emotional regulation, a culmination of all development in the first year and a harbinger of the self-regulation that is to come" (p. 172). Thus the quality of attachment is an important aspect of developmental risk and resiliency. Children with access to stable and nurturing primary relationships can experience and successfully regulate wider ranges of affect. Children without access, or with uneven access, to such relationships are more likely to show developmental deficits in the regulation of affect and, relatedly, in the capacity to engage in exploratory play.

The "Strange Situation" (Ainsworth et al., 1978) is an experimental procedure that has been used to observe the internal working model of infants and to classify patterns of attachment between infants and their primary caregivers. Infants are observed as they explore a new play situation, interact with a friendly stranger, and experience a separation from, and reunion with, their primary caregiver. Researchers are trained to observe the ways in which infants (1) seek out proximity to their caregivers, (2) experience distress when separated from their caregivers, and (3) utilize caregivers as a secure base and source of comfort when distressed.

The Strange Situation technique has resulted in the identification of four distinct patterns of "secure" or "insecure" attachment (Cassidy & Shaver, 1999). Each pattern of attachment is presumed to reflect the quality of infant–caregiver interaction and the degree to which the caregiver supports the developing infant's sense of security and capacity for exploration. Although a full explication of these attachment patterns is beyond the scope of this chapter, more in-depth reviews are available elsewhere (Cassidy & Shaver, 1999). Below we briefly define each attachment pattern, with particular emphasis on how early relational experience either supports or impedes the developing child's capacity to experience affect alone, to share affect in a relational context, and to regulate states of affective arousal both independently and in concert with a primary caregiver.

SECURE ATTACHMENT

Infants categorized as "securely attached" are able to seek out and utilize proximity to the caregiver when distressed and are able to utilize the caregiver as a secure base from which to explore and gain mastery over the external world. Although secure infants may be upset at separation from the caregiver, they are characterized by their ability to regain homeostasis and resume other activities, such as play and exploration, upon the caregiver's return. In addition, securely attached infants are likely to utilize strategies such as "social referencing" or "checking back" with the caregiver when exploring a new toy or experience. These behaviors provide opportunities for affective sharing between infant and caregiver and provide the infant with important information about the caregiver's broader experience and judgment. For example, an infant approaching a new toy, who "checks back" with the caregiver in a bid to share his or her excitement, may also receive important signals that draw his or her attention to particular details of the toy (e.g., "Look! It makes music!"), to potentially dangerous aspects of the situation (e.g., "Hmm . . . that toy looks sharp. Here . . . let me give you another toy to play with"), or to the infant's own emotional experience of the situation (e.g., "You like the music in that toy, don't you?"). In these examples, a secure attachment pattern not only promotes proximity and exploration, but also embedded are processes of affective sharing and opportunities for the infant to learn from the parent's experience.

"Insecure" or "anxious" attachments represent infant–caregiver dyads that are not consistently organized to achieve the dual goals of security and exploration. Classified as "insecure/avoidant," "insecure/resistant," or "disorganized," these attachment patterns are associated with a range of suboptimal developmental outcomes involving difficulties in the regulation of affective arousal, interpersonal interaction, and the capacity for cognitive attention in a range of settings. It has been through observation of insecure attachment patterns that researchers and clinicians have had the greatest opportunity to consider the role of secure attachment in the developing child's emerging capacity for affect regulation.

Insecure/Avoidant Attachment "Insecure/avoidant" infants may, on the surface, appear to be less anxious in novel surroundings or when separated from the caregiver. In addition, they are not as likely to seek out the caregiver following separation *or* to use the caregiver as a secure base by "checking back" with him or her before approaching a new person or toy. These infants, even while in the company of caregivers and others, may appear to "play alone" and to remain somewhat oblivious to the emotional stance or reaction of others. As we discuss below, infants classified as insecure/avoidant may have learned, via repeated interactions with primary caregivers, that dyadic interaction is not associated with positive affective experiences. These infants have developed a style of early "reliance on the self" that may place them at risk primarily because they do not have as many opportunities to benefit from adult judgment and experience. These infants may modulate their own experience by appearing more "shut down." At times, caregivers will describe these infants as "so good . . . they never ask for anything." Day-care providers might describe these infants as "easy" or "nondemanding." And yet, these infants are likely to be missing out on important developmental opportunities. The insecure/avoidant infant is more likely, as a toddler, to be in a situation of danger resulting from an absence of reliance on adults. For example, a child who is avoidantly attached may act on his or her own impulses without "checking in" with an adult. Such a child may wander off or away from caregivers as opposed to communicating his or her desires (e.g., "I go out-side") or expressing a wish for a shared experience (e.g., "Mommy, come with me?").

Insecure/Resistant Attachment Infants classified as "insecure/resistant" display the greatest degree of distress in the Strange Situation. These infants tend to be highly distressed upon separation from their caregivers and not as likely to be able to utilize the caregivers as a secure base from which to explore a new environment. While insecure/resistant infants are highly distressed at separation, they are not as able as securely attached infants to rely on the presence of the caregiver to regain a state of homeostasis. Upon reunion with caregivers, insecure/resistant infants may seek out contact but then show varying patterns of resistance, such as turning away, stiffening their arms and not accepting an embrace, and most importantly, not being able to use the caregivers to modulate negative affect sufficiently to return to the important activities of play and exploration.

Disorganized Attachment Infants classified as "disorganized" show the greatest insecurity in that their attachment behavior is observed to be confused and inconsistent (Solomon & George, 1999). This pattern of attachment is overrepresented among groups of infants and young children who have experienced chronic abuse and neglect (Shields & Cicchetti, 2001). When a supportive relational environment does not exist or the attachment relationship has been disrupted, the infant may experience severe stress and develop behavioral mechanisms for coping with poorly regulated interactive experiences (Cassidy & Shaver, 1999). In her seminal work in the field of infant mental health, Selma Fraiberg and her colleagues (Fraiberg, 1980) described the emergence of infant defenses such as gaze aversion, withdrawal, aggression against the self, hyperactivity, lethargy, and extreme separation anxiety. Although these defenses may temporarily function to relieve internal states of anxiety of affective dysregulation, they clearly limit the infant's developmental opportunities in other ways. Such infants and young children may be impaired in important capacities related to affect regulation, such as the ability to self-soothe, to achieve sufficient homeostasis so that other cognitive tasks (e.g., problem solving) can be approached, to articulate feeling states, or, as development proceeds, to utilize language and important relationships (both inside and outside the family) to modify their emotional lives and experiences in a therapeutic manner. The following points summarize the information in this section:

- Patterns of attachment reflect differences in the success of caregiver–infant dyads in achieving the dual developmental goals of security and exploration.
- Attachment has been empirically measured by assessing infant behavior in laboratory conditions (the Strange Situation) that present infants with a new environment, new people, and brief separation from caregivers.
- Of particular interest are the infant's capacity (1) to utilize the caregiver as a secure base for exploration, (2) to seek out proximity to caregiver when distressed, and (3) to effectively utilize the caregiver in the elaboration of positive, and the modulation of negative, affective experiences.
- 'Four attachment patterns have been identified.' These are secure, insecure/avoidant, insecure/anxious, and disorganized.

Developmental Consequences of Attachment Patterns

The quality of attachment between infants and their primary caregivers has emerged as an important determinant of risk and resiliency in infancy and across maturational phases of development (Lieberman & Zeanah, 1995; Main and Goldwyn, 1991). Clinicians often come into contact with children whose attachment histories are characterized by separations, losses, or exposure to inconsistent, neglectful, or abusive care. Such children represent an "at-risk" group, whose presenting problems can be better understood in terms of the developmental consequences of attachment experiences. A knowledge base of this information can inform assessment and intervention as well as help clinicians to understand their role as a new relational partner for the child (Shapiro, Shapiro, & Paret, 2001).

From a variety of theoretical perspectives, studies have shown that early caregiving that is characterized by warmth, sensitivity, empathy, and contingent responsiveness is associated with a secure attachment pattern and a range of positive outcomes in social, cognitive, emotional, and physical spheres of development (Ainsworth, Blehar, Waters, & Wall, 1978). In contrast, infants and young children who do not have access to stable and empathic relationships are at risk for a range of developmental problems both in infancy and across time (Carlson, 1998; Erickson, Sroufe, & Egeland, 1985). Research in the cognitive neurosciences has identified neurobiological correlates of early caregiving that provide insight into the mechanisms by which early relational experiences, such as those comprising "attachment," shape aspects of the child's nervous system and are associated with the child's ability to cope with stress and regulate other affective states (Gunnar, 2001; Ito, Teicher, Glod, & Ackerman, 1998).

Infants classified as securely attached are more likely than those classified as insecure or disorganized (1) to be socially competent, (2) to be active problem solvers, (3) to show mastery motivation, (4) to be empathic with others, (5) to make and sustain friendships, (6) to be able to rely on noncaregiring adults when necessary, and (7) to be able to regulate affective states in developmentally appropriate and adaptive ways. Conversely, infants classified as insecure or disorganized are more likely to show evidence of some level of psychopathology as development continues. Among the clinical outcomes observed are difficulties in the regulation of affect and emotion, a higher incidence of antisocial behavior, and lower levels of empathic understanding. Longitudinal studies on attachment describe powerful associations between early attachment quality and longer-term indicators of emotional well-being—not only in childhood, but through adolescence and adulthood as well (George, Kaplan, & Main, 1996; Lieberman & Pawl, 1990; Sroufe, Egeland, & Kreutzer, 1990).

An important focus of research is the effort to understand the biopsychosocial *processes* by which early attachment experiences affect later developmental well-being. Understanding the causal pathway between early relational experience, or attachment, and later indices of social and emotional well-being is critical in helping clinicians to identify important aspects of risk and resiliency. Researchers have focused both on the normative case, as when the adults, as children, had access to stable and empathic care, and the more atypical case, as when individuals were exposed to inconsistent, neglectful, or traumatic caregiving in early life (Perry, 1994).

The study of how early attachment affects later developmental outcomes is an important nexus of developmental and neuroscience research (Carlson & Earls, 1997; Dawson, Frey, & Panagiotides, 1997; Schore, 1997a). These fields of study converge on the importance of early attachments because early brain development is, in part, dependent on the quality of interpersonal experience. As is the case with the formation of attachment bonds, a sensitive period exists during the first several years of life for those aspects of brain development thought to underlie important aspects of emotional development, such as the capacity for affect regulation.

What causes different patterns of attachment to develop? Why are some babies securely attached whereas others display insecure/anxious, insecure/avoidant, or disorganized patterns of attachment? Research on attachment has shown that security of attachment is based on a combination of factors that includes caregiver characteristics, infant characteristics, and a range of contextual factors (Belsky, 1984). Of particular interest to researchers and clinicians is the role of parenting behavior as a determining factor of attachment quality in infancy and early childhood.

Infants who are securely attached are more likely to have caregivers who are emotionally available, able to respond empathically to the needs of the child, and able to engage in affectively attuned interactions as the child experiences both positive and negative states of psychophysiological arousal. "Keeping the child in mind," recognizing the importance of caregiving, and understanding the child's internal world are central components of adults who foster secure attachments (Winnicott, 1965d). Siegel (1999) referred to such caregivers us having "mindsight," the capacity to understand the mind of the other. Caregivers who are able to accurately perceive and reflect the emotional world of the child are more able to respond with sensitivity and empathy (Fonagy, Steele, Moran, Steele, & Higgit, 1991). Caregivers who are able to reflect on the child's experience and on their own internal state are more able to help the child learn that even negative states of emotion are tolerable, and that it is possible to return to a state of homeostatic balance. This understanding may, in turn, contribute to the formation of a more optimistic sense of self. Thus a "secure attachment" describes a caregiving relationship that protects the child from being overwhelmed by negative affect *and* enables the child to rely on the caregiver as an "auxiliary ego," thereby augmenting the child's ability to regulate affect and engage in learning and relationships.

The relationship between attachment classification and psychopathology is being examined as more longitudinal studies on attachment are completed. Many studies have noted the association between patterns of insecure attachment and behavior problems in preschool children (Erickson et al., 1985). These problems are exacerbated when other risk factors (e.g., poverty) are present. Through the development of a structured interview (Fonagy et al., 1995; George, Kaplan, & Main, 1996), it has become possible to empirically assess the degree of continuity of attachment classification from infancy through adolescence and adulthood. By examining such data in conjunction with additional data on personality and indicators of mental health, it is possible to empirically test the relationship between early attachment classifications, later classification of attachment style, and indices of mental health and illness.

The Intergenerational Transmission of Attachment Patterns: Reflective Functioning and Mentalization

Longitudinal research on attachment suggests that caregivers' internal representations of their own attachment experiences are strongly associated with the quality of attachment that forms between them and their infants. The ability of adult caregivers to provide the reflective and empathic care associated with secure attachment formation is related to caregivers' internal representations of their own early attachment experiences (Cassidy & Shaver, 1999) Research on the intergenerational transmission of attachment patterns suggests that the capacity for empathy, marked by a reflective and intentional stance toward the infant, is a cornerstone of sensitive parenting, strongly associated with secure attachment, and a partial consequence of the adult's own attachment history

(Fonagy, Steele, & Steele, 1991; Steele, Steele, & Fonagy, 1996). This research is important because it moves beyond the more traditional notion of sensitivity to describe the psychological basis of the parent's ability to engage in the formation of attachment bonds.

Steele, Steele, and Fonagy (1996) pointed out that standard measures of parental sensitivity are not sufficient to explain observed continuity in the intergenerational transmission of attachment patterns. Indeed, other researchers have also made efforts to "unpack" the construct of attachment and define more specifically the psychological elements that enable caregivers to be empathic, attuned, and contingently responsive to the infants and children in their care (Emde, 1985; Stern, 1985; Winnicott, 1965d). This work is extremely important because it helps clinicians and researchers to envision how the attachment relationship may *change form* over time *while maintaining psychological continuity*, infused with the parent's understanding of the child's emerging psychological self and emotional world.

Winnicott (1965d) introduced the concept of the "holding environment" to describe the context of care that envelops the infant and young child. The "good-enough" holding environment described by Winnicott is characterized *not* by perfect synchrony and sensitivity between parent and infant, but by caregiving that is globally stable, consistent, reflective of the infant's emerging needs, and infused with an understanding of the infant's emotional life and development. The construct of the holding environment is particularly useful in considering how the function of parent–infant attachment must evolve as the child's development proceeds in many spheres.

The "holding" of the infant initially refers, in part, to the physical holding and caregiving provided to support the infant's modulation of physiological states such as hunger, the need for warmth, and the regulation of sleep–wake cycles and states of alertness. Quickly, though, development proceeds, and the concept of holding broadens to include the parent's role in containing and reflecting the emergence of the child's psychological self in the context of the attachment relationship. This is a complex task; as the child develops, he or she may come to express a broad range of feelings that evokes varied responses in the adults responsible for his or her care. A parent's ability to recognize and accept the broadest range of a child's feelings, including anxiety and other negative affective states, is central to the parent's ability to provide supportive care.

When the attachment relationship develops within a good-enough holding environment, the caregiver is able to help the infant modulate affect in ways that sustain the infant's psychic investment in interpersonal relationships and, ultimately, support the child's emerging capacities for self-soothing. When a supportive environment does not exist and the child does not have the experience of being psychologically held, he or she may develop defenses to guard against the psychic pain associated with overwhelming affective states or interpersonal experiences that are either understimulating (e.g., neglect) or overstimulating and intrusive (Fonagy & Target, 1998).

Early studies in the field of infant mental health (Fraiberg, 1980) described the coping mechanisms of children who are unable to rely on the auxiliary support of the caregiver for the developmentally appropriate regulation of affective arousal. Such infants may exhibit behavioral patterns of withdrawal, freezing, physical aggression or marked disorganization in their relational interactions. It is important that clinicians learn to recognize such behaviors as potential indicators of difficulties in the caregiving environment and as adaptations children may have made in response to psychologically painful relational experiences (Shapiro et al., 2001; Paret & Shapiro, 1998). In the following chapters on vulnerable dyads and infant mental health, examples demonstrate how clinicians are utilizing these concepts to inform the work of assessment and treatment.

Why are some parents better able to provide empathic care that reflects the child's internal world and emotional needs? As we have seen, studies on the intergenerational transmission of attachment patterns have addressed this question by focusing on specific metacognitive capacities, such as the ability to reflect on and mentalize, or think about, the internal thoughts and states of others (Steele, Steele, & Fonagy, 1996). "Reflective function" refers to the cognitive and emotional capacities that enable a parent to "understand that her own or another's behaviors are linked in meaningful, predictable ways to underlying mental states, to feelings, wishes, thoughts and desires" (Slade, 2002, p. 11). Individuals who are high in reflective function are able to understand the symbolic and emotional substrate of behavior. Relatedly, reflective functioning enables the individual to think about, or mentalize, the nature of other people's experiences and behaviors. In this way, reflective function provides a way to create a "mental model" (Slade, 2002) of the other's experience. Reflective functioning and the related capacity for mentalization support sensitive parenting and attachment security because they allow the caregiver to understand the meaning and emotional nature of the child's expressions and behaviors, thereby enabling the caregiver to respond not only to the child's physical needs but to his or her emotional needs as well. In addition, the ability to reflect on and mentalize about one's own feelings and those of the child help the child "make meaning of feelings and internal experiences states of psychophysiological arousal associated with feelings without becoming overwhelmed and shutting down" (Slade, 2002, p. 11). Thus reflective function and the capacity for mentalization are closely tied to the genesis of the capacity for affect regulation—itself a cornerstone and consequence of the attachment relationship.

PSYCHOSOCIAL EFFECTS OF EARLY RELATIONAL DEPRIVATION

The field of developmental psychopathology is concerned with the study of "normal" and "abnormal" development. From this perspective, clinical research on "at-risk populations" has much to contribute to our understanding of "normal" or "expected" pathways of development.

The conceptual frame of developmental psychopathology has provided an important framework for studying the development of children without access to stable attachment relationships and/or children whose attachments are characterized by abuse and neglect (Cicchetti & Cohen, 1995). These studies have been very generative in terms of our understanding of the processes by which early relational care impacts development and of the degree of plasticity, or capacity to recover, following experiences of traumatic, disorganized or neglectful care. Below is a brief summary on the psychosocial effects of early relational deprivation, followed by a discussion of the impact of such deprivation on central aspects of early neurobiological development.

The absence of stable and high-quality attachment bonds constitutes deprivation for the infant and young child. While researchers agree that relational deprivation creates vulnerability and risk for the infant and young child, it is also true that experiences of deprivation may be qualitatively different and thus may have differential effects on developmental well-being (Paret & Shapiro, 1998; Shapiro et al., 2001; Webb, 1996). As Gunnar, Bruce, and Grotevant (2001) pointed out, deprivation may be characterized by a lack of access to health care and nutrition, a lack of age-appropriate stimulation and opportunities for learning, and most importantly from our perspective on attachment, by a lack of access to stable and responsive relationships. As is true of many risk factors, the experience of one "kind" of deprivation is likely to be associated with others as well. For example, infants without access to stable relationships may be less likely to have access to appropriate kinds of sensory stimulation.

Studies on early deprivation have focused on a range of developmental outcomes. Researchers have examined the effects of deprivation on intelligence and cognitive development, language development, physical growth, and social and emotional development. Overall, these studies have suggested that although all areas of early development are affected by deprivation, when a more enriched environment is provided, many aspects of cognitive, language, and physical development may "catch up" (Gunnar, 2001). More nuanced aspects of social and emotional development, many of which have cognitive elements, are not only directly affected by experiences of deprivation but are more likely to persist even after the child's relational environment improves (if it does). Among the developmental risks observed are an increased reactivity to stress, problems with the regulation of affect and anxiety, difficulty in the areas of impulse control, and ongoing difficulties in the formation of new attachment bonds with caregivers and peers.

Research on the effects of early relational deprivation on the social and emotional development of children is extremely important for clinicians who work with children who have experienced disruption or trauma in their early caregiving relationships. In these cases, the child's "developmental" age may be much younger than his or her chronological age, and the parents may need intensive support in their efforts to engage and sustain the child in the attachment relationship. In particular, parents may need assistance in becoming sensitive, reflective observers of their child's emotional signals and needs, because the child's behavior may be defensively organized to withdraw from interaction or to resist efforts at engagement.

Infants and young children who have lacked access to reflective care may exhibit marked deficits in their ability to mentalize their own emotional world and the feelings and intentions of other people. Many clinicians have worked with children who consistently make inaccurate attributions about the meaning of other people's behavior, leading them to see aggression where none was intended, or leaving them unable to "read" the social cues and needs of other people. Children who have not had the opportunity to develop a sense of trust with known caregivers may find it difficult to rely on adults or to believe themselves valued by caregivers. Defensively, these children may reject new offers of love and concern and may show great difficulty in the modulation of anxiety and other affective states.

When children lack the capacity for reflection and have difficulties in mentalizing the experience of others, they are not prepared to empathically engage with other people. To the extent that impaired reflective functioning is associated with problems in attachment, so too are a lack of empathy for the feelings of others and poor impulse control (Perry, 2004). Lack of empathy combines with problems in impulsivity to create difficulties in the modulation of aggression toward others. Indeed, a common problem observed among children with traumatic attachment histories is the propensity to act aggressively against others, with no genuine feelings of remorse for the pain caused (Perry, 2004). Researchers believe this lack of remorse to be a consequence of an incapacity for empathic understanding of others' mental states.

THE PSYCHOBIOLOGY OF AFFECTIVE ATTUNEMENT:
ATTACHMENT AND BRAIN DEVELOPMENT

In Chapter 1 we reviewed research on the nature of brain development in early life. In this section we turn our attention to research on the neurobiological correlates of attachment. Attachment research is an important conceptual framework for the study of early brain development because researchers have identified the quality of early interpersonal experience as a primary "environmental" determinant of brain development in early life. In conjunction with access to health and nutrition and the absence of abuse and neglect, the quality of early care, culminating in the formation of attachment bonds, impacts many processes of brain development and, in turn, affects the neurobiological substrate of the capacity for affect regulation and the ability to mediate exposure to stress in ways that protect adaptive capacity (Gunnar, Brodersen, Nachmias, Buss, & Rigatuso, 1996; Shonkoff & Phillips, 2000).

Just as researchers have studied the developmental course of attachment in the first few years of life, so too have researchers explored the developmental course of early brain development. This research has produced an understanding of the first few years of life as a "sensitive" period in brain development (Nelson & Bloom, 1997). Although brain development continues across the lifespan, the first few years of life represent particular moments of developmental opportunity for those aspects of synaptic formation that are strongly shaped by the quality of experience, that is, the nature of early caregiving (Greenough & Black, 1992).

Schore (1994, 2000) described the processes by which attuned, sensitive caregiver–infant interaction supports aspects of early brain development that are associated with social and emotional competency. He stated that during periods of infant-caregiver attunement, there is right brain to right brain communication during which both partners express and process emotional information. An empathically attuned caregiver regulates his or her own affect and *also* reflects back to the child a model of affect regulation. Given that infancy and early childhood are critical developmental periods for neural circuitry, the regulation of stress-related hormones is critical.

Brain development in early life proceeds from the simple to the more complex, from the "lower" to the "higher" regions of the brain. How higher areas of the right brain develop is an important focus of research because these parts of the brain provide the neurobiological substrate for key aspects of social and emotional adaptive capacities. Research has shown that the more complex areas of the right brain are "involved in empathically reading the faces, voices and gestures of other humans, in appraising bodily responses to such social stimuli, in regulating resultant emotional states, and in coping with internal and external stress" (Schore, 2000, p. 1). That the right brain develops in the context of early interpersonal experience provides a connection between the more familiar understanding of how the capacity for empathy and affect regulation results from contingently responsive caregiving and new studies that describe how such caregiving shapes neuronal circuitry, the development of memory, and aspects of neurochemistry associated with the mediation of stress responses (Gunnar, 2000).

Bowlby's construct of the internal working model is being examined anew in the context of research on early brain development. Specifically, the idea that a child develops an internal mental representation of a co-constructed attachment relationship requires an understanding of how children form and store preverbal and other kinds of memory. Research on brain development has shed new light on the nature of memory, differentiating types of memory such as "implicit" and "explicit." The internal working model represents an implicit memory, most likely at the unconscious level, of the attachment relationship. As an implicit memory, the internal working model is stored in the right hemisphere of the brain and acts as a substrate of the child's expectations as to whether his or her needs will be met and whether states of affective arousal will be calmed or become implicit signals that overwhelming anxiety and dysregulation are to follow. Clinicians may be familiar with the behavior of anxiously attached children who vigilantly attend to caregiver signals and may respond to even slight facial or nonverbal gestures as preludes to impending disorganization or overwhelming anxiety. Such behaviors are evidence of the child's internal working model, or implicit memories of attachment, at work and are relevant to many contexts (e.g., child welfare) in which clinicians must make rapid assessments and intervention plans.

Decades of multidisciplinary research on attachment combine to highlight the importance of primary attachment relationships as critical elements in the child's developing capacities for the experience and regulation of affective states. Individual differences in the quality of attachment, as measured by "security" and "insecurity," are associated with a range of important developmental outcomes. As research in the cognitive neurosciences proceeds, an important focus is the exploration of the neurobiological substrate of patterns of attachment. Specifically, researchers are interested in (1) the processes of physiological and neurobiological regulation in the infant, (2) the role of the caregiver as a coregulator of the infant's experience, (3) environmental contributions to parent–infant regulatory capacities, and (4) the ways in which early relational development and experiences shape the neurobiological substrate of emotional well-being.

As research in the cognitive neurosciences continues to provide increased clarity on the ways in which early relational experience, or attachment relationships, affect the child's developing capacity for emotional regulation, researchers and clinicians alike are focusing anew on the determinants and consequences of attachment quality as predictors of mental health outcomes in children and adults. Beyond infancy and early childhood, the quality of attachment relationships is often inferred by observating the pattern of relating between individuals and others. In his or her pattern of affiliation, does an individual show an ability to trust other people and a sense of constancy with regard to primary relationships? Alternatively, does an individual find affiliation with others to be primarily anxiety provoking or otherwise psychologically unsettling? In the therapeutic context, it is important to note if the client faces internal obstacles to engaging with the practitioner that might be related to earlier relational experiences, either within the client's family or in past professional helping relationships. Additionally, themes related to attachment are often important in clinical work with both children and adults. It is important that practitioners listen for these themes in the narratives of their clients so that important opportunities for engagement and intervention are not lost.

The relationship between early attachment quality and later mental health outcomes is mediated, in part, by the presence or absence of other relational opportunities with caregivers, peers, and other interested adults (Perry, 1995). This is an important point because one of the most salient findings in the study of the neuroscience of emotional development is the fact that the developing brain remains open to new experience, at least to some degree, across the lifespan. Thus, although certain periods of time are more sensitive or critical in terms of emotional and relational development, the advent of new experiences and relationships may make both positive and negative contributions to the neurobiology of mental health across time. This last finding is particularly salient to the practice of developmentally informed psychotherapy, which focuses on the ways in which therapeutically informed relational experiences can provide important avenues of support and growth for children and their families.

Chapter 6

VULNERABLE DYADS

The Quality of Early Caregiving Relationships

THE INTERPERSONAL EXPERIENCE of the infant is an important developmental context for social, emotional, physical, and cognitive growth (Stern, 1985). The emergence, during the first year of life, of the attachment relationship is a reflection of the countless interactions that have occurred between the infant and primary caregivers during this period of rapid development and growth.

Research on attachment has shown that the quality of parent–infant attachment is related to multiple developmental competencies that emerge over time (Page, 2000). Children that are cared for in a sensitive, emotionally attuned manner are more likely to develop internal working models that reflect the expectation that caregivers are trustworthy and will behave in a developmentally supportive way that buttresses the child's emerging capacity to regulate states of arousal and affect. A secure internal working model of attachment is also associated with the child's sense that he or she is worthy of this kind of care (Main & Goldwyn, 1991). As they grow older, securely attached children are able, having internalized a positive image of the caregiver, to turn their attention confidently to the larger object world of people and exploration.

The developmental benefit of a "secure" internal working model of attachment is evident in the child's ability to sustain investment in the external world of objects and people and, over time, to experience an increasingly broad range of affect (Greenspan & Porges, 1984). In addition, the child's capacity to achieve a "good-enough" capacity to regulate affect is also strongly shaped by the degree to which the caregiver is able, over time, to accurately perceive the child's internal state and overt expressions of emotion, *and* the degree to which the caregiver is able to respond in an empathically attuned manner.

CASE EXAMPLES

Consider the following brief vignettes that describe the combination of environmental and psychosocial stress that young children and their caregivers may face as they traverse the early years of parenting and child development. The clinical implications of these contexts, in terms of assessment and intervention, are discussed more fully in Chapter 7.

Tanya: Secure Attachment Despite Economic Stress

Tanya was first seen by a social worker at the age of 12 months, when her family was being evaluated at a family service agency. Although under a great deal of economic stress, Tanya's mother has been able to provide emotional stability for her young child. Believing that communication with Tanya is important, her mother uses language to "explain" daily routines to Tanya and also to put into words what she, the mother, is observing about Tanya. For example, when a "stranger" walked into the waiting room and Tanya furrowed her brow and looked toward her mother, her mother responded, "What happened, T? Did someone you don't know walk into the room?" Similarly, when Tanya found a toy that she liked and squealed with delight, her mother responded, "Wow, I can tell that you really like that toy, right, T?" Tanya's mother maintained her emotional availability to Tanya even as she sat across the room from her and was asked to fill out forms for the purpose of the office visit. It would have been easy for an observer to tell, even in a crowded waiting room, that Tanya and her mother were a dyad. While Tanya showed interest in other people, it was her mother with whom she "checked back" when she felt any uncertainty or when she was looking to share positive affect.

Michael: Lacking a Sense of Connection Even in Situational Stability

At the time of this observation, Michael was 17 months old. Since his birth, Michael has been in three different foster homes, having been returned once, and then removed again, from the care of his biological mother. Michael was observed playing with age-appropriate toys in the middle of a playroom. Although showing some interest in toys by picking them up and putting them down, his play was rather "flat" in that he appeared to take little interest in any particular toy. Moreover, Michael made no effort to "share" his discoveries via eye contact with his foster mother or with the examiner. He played quietly, and as his foster mother observed, is a "very good toddler"—almost as if "he doesn't need attention." Even when the foster mother had to leave the room momentarily, Michael seemed not to notice and certainly displayed no anxiety or uncomfortable affect. Nor did he show any visible response upon her return. His foster mother commented, "It's like he's here alone . . . I don't know if he would notice if I weren't here."

VULNERABLE DYADS

Many parent–child dyads are deemed "vulnerable" because various risk factors, or sets of factors, combine to inhibit the caregiver's ability to accurately perceive or respond to the emotional or physical needs of the developing child. In addition to a range of contextual and social factors, such as social isolation and poverty, other factors may interfere with (1) the caregiver's own capacity for emotion regulation, (2) the ability to take the point of view of the child, and (3) the ability to use language to represent either his or her own emotional experience or to reflect back to the child the parental perception of the child's internal state of mind and experience. These kinds of obstacles interfere with the child's developing sense of "being known" or "understood" by the caregiver, resulting in critical problems in the child's emerging capacity to identify affective states, relate particular states of affect to known experience, and to regulate affect in a manner sufficient to help the child reinstate homeostasis when his or her affective experience becomes dysregulated.

As has been discussed elsewhere in this volume, the relational environment of infants and young children is a primary context for early brain development. Because early brain development is experience- or use-dependent, children whose early caregiving is compromised by emotional or physical deprivation are at risk (Perry, Pollard, Blakely, Baker, & Vigilante, 1995). The developing brain "stores" information depending, in part, on which neuronal connections are "activated" most often (Perry et al. 1995). One of the reasons that researchers describe the early years as a "critical" or "sensitive" period with regard to brain development is because both the organization and function of the child's neural systems are so affected during this time by the *amount* and *quality* of interactive experience. In particular, human infants are uniquely dependent on their adult caregivers for the provision of an environment that provides sufficient contingent responsivity (Gunnar, 1998).

Many studies have documented the effects of inadequate caregiving on various aspects of brain development (Nelson & Bloom, 1997). These studies highlight the need for initial and early intervention for "at-risk" parents and children (Olds, Eckenrode, & Henderson, 1997). These studies also suggest that although brain development retains plasticity over time, some effects of early neglect and disrupted caregiving may continue to exert influence on child development and behavior, via their impact on brain development, even after situational stability has been attained (Perry, 1995; Hofer, 1995; Shapiro & Applegate, 2000).

Models of risk and resiliency are used as a conceptual foundation for the development of preventive and tertiary care interventions for parents and children defined as being "at risk" for negative developmental outcomes. In order to infuse these efforts with more clinical meaning, it is important to further specify the broad categorization of being at risk. If certain groups of parent–child dyads are labeled "at developmental risk," important questions emerge. Consider the following:

- For what particular negative developmental outcomes is this group at "risk"?
- Are all members of the group at the same level of developmental risk? Why or why not?
- What factors have been identified that combine to place a particular group at risk?
- What are the processes by which "risk factors" operate?

These kinds of questions are central to models of risk and resiliency and thus provide an important foundation for the development of *nuanced* assessment, prevention, and intervention strategies.

In this chapter we consider several at-risk groups of parents and children. Adolescent parenthood, maternal depression, and parental drug abuse are commonly recognized as serious risks to child and family development. Considered at risk for many social, psychological, physical, and developmental reasons, these groups can each be examined in terms of a variety of risk factors that can affect the parent–child relationship in ways that impair the quality of attachment and important developmental outcomes. Familiar from a psychosocial perspective, we seek to apply the research reviewed earlier in this text that discusses the connections between caregiver–child interaction patterns, the quality of attachment that emerges, and the related neurobiological development of children in early life. As previously noted, research on brain development and attachment shows that impaired early relational experience can create psychological and neurobiological vulnerability in the child that is sustained over time (Lott, 1998). Additionally, this research sharpens our understanding of how psychological and developmental vulnerability in a caregiver can be "transferred", from parent to child, and sustained across generations (Fraiberg, 1980; Muir, 1992; Schore, 1996; Weatherston, 2000).

Our work in this chapter begins with a discussion of how parenting behavior is understood, from a multidisciplinary perspective, as an important mediator of child development outcomes. Many models of developmental risk in childhood focus on those factors that affect the quality of parenting behavior, which, in turn, shapes the developmental experience of the child (Belsky, 1984). As we have discussed elsewhere in this volume, disruptions in early caregiving experience are among the most damaging kinds of "stress" experienced by infants and young children. Thus, we continue our discussion with a brief review of literature on the experience of stress in early life and the ways in which the neurobiological changes that accompany sustained stress may create additional vulnerability for already at-risk young children.

PARENTING BEHAVIOR AS A MEDIATOR
OF CHILD WELL-BEING

Researchers have described the importance of parenting, or the caregiving context, as a determinant of child well-being from a variety of theoretical perspectives (Ainsworth et al., 1978; Bowlby, 1969; Steele, Steele, Croft, & Fonagy, 1999; Stern, 1985; Winnicott, 1965d). A rich multidisciplinary literature highlights the importance of parental behavior to a range of child development outcomes. This work includes studies of attachment processes (Ainsworth et al., 1978), early childhood education (Shonkoff & Phillips, 2000), and early social and emotional development (Schore, 1994; Shapiro & Applegate, 2000; Stern, 1985).

Research on attachment and, more generally, research on the quality of interaction between children and their caregivers, has expanded our understanding of the importance of positive early care. This knowledge base can help practitioners assess at-risk parent–child dyads and provide more informed primary, secondary, and tertiary care (Shapiro et al., 2001). The quality of caregiver–child interactions, sometimes indexed by a measurement of attachment security, is associated with a range of developmental outcomes in cognitive, social, physical, and emotional spheres of development (Cassidy & Shaver, 1999). Parenting behavior associated with secure attachment and with more optimal child outcomes is often characterized as warm, sensitive, contingently responsive, empathic, and at-tuned (Ainsworth et al., 1978; Stern, 1985).

Many factors may interfere with the capacity for sensitive parenting behavior, including (1) lack of knowledge about child development; (2) depression or other cognitive–affective disturbances that impair the parent's ability to interpret infant signals; (3) an inability to put the needs of another ahead of one's own; (4) lack of identification with the mater-nal role; (5) unresolved conflicts over dependency; (6) high levels of stress, and (7) low levels of social support.

Researchers have developed models of parenting behavior in an effort to identify factors associated with variations in parenting competence (Belsky, 1984). Such models identify factors that either facilitate or impede optimal parenting behavior and, relatedly, child development outcomes. Generally speaking, process models of parenthood focus on three interrelated sets of factors that may combine to shape parenting behavior: (1) the psychologi-cal health and well-being of the parent, (2) structural sources of stress and support, and (3) a confluence of important child characteristics, such as health and neurophysiological status (Beckwith, 1990; Phillips & Shon-koff, 2001). This kind of process model is useful in conceptualizing those groups of parents and children who may be at risk or vulnerable due to fac-tors that fall into one or more of the above groups.

HOW NEUROSCIENCE SUPPORTS EXISTING PSYCHOSOCIAL MODELS

Psychosocial models of early development have been supported by new research in neuroscience that helps us to understand how the nature of early relational experience affects the developing organization and struc-ture of the brain (Dawson et al., 1992; Schore, 1997a; Shapiro & Apple-gate, 2000). This research has helped to refocus our understanding so that we no longer think of "nature" and "nurture" as dichotomous variables, but can understand the unfolding of a child's genetic potential *through* the child's experience of nurturance. Neurobiological factors are intertwined with early relational experience.

Many groups of at-risk parents and children are characterized by atypical patterns of interaction and disruptions in early caregiving relationships. Research in the cognitive neurosciences has provided a new window into the clinical meaning of disorganized or traumatic early care experiences by delineating how disrupted early care precipitates change in the early wiring of the brain: in neurobiological and neurochemical processes that have import for the experience and regulation of affect. Thus any factors or set of characteristics that are associated with the parental capacity for affect regulation or the child's developing capacity to regulate affect are understood as appropriate targets for support and intervention.

As we have described elsewhere in this volume, the early years of life represent a highly sensitive period with regard to brain development and, in particular, with regard to the influence of caregiving experience on brain organization, structure, and function (Nelson & Bloom, 1997). It is now well understood that the human brain triples in size by 3 years of age and that the first year of life is a critical period with regard to the development of the prefrontal cortex, a part of the brain that is an important element of the biological basis of attachment behavior. As Dawson and Colleagues (1992) and Schore (1996) have pointed out, the early years of life are also a critical time because of the dominance of the right hemisphere of the brain during the infancy and early childhood. Research in affective neuroscience has clearly shown that early attachment and caregiving patterns directly influence the development of the frontal limbic system in the brain's right hemisphere.

When children lack access to an enriched environment or experience significant disruptions in early caregiving, their ability to achieve homeostasis and to become self-regulating is impaired. Through the use of animal models, researchers have begun to conceptualize how experiences of early neglect and disruption in attachment relationships precipitate neurobiological changes that may persist even if the child's relational environment improves (Perry et al., 1995). Studies on the neurobiological effects of disrupted care and relational stress are important from a clinical perspective because they show how stress-related neurobiological changes may underlie psychosocial clinical symptoms. In addition, these studies help to explain why children who experience disruptions in early care may remain vulnerable to new stresses as they appear later in life.

THE NEUROBIOLOGY OF CHILDHOOD STRESS

In all children, stress precipitates several kinds of biological changes. In mild forms, these psychophysiological changes are important signals that may help the child to mobilize adaptive coping responses. These biological changes occur in the amygdala, hippocampus, hypothalamus, pituitary gland, and adrenal cortex. Measurable biological responses to stress include the release of adrenalin, stimulation of the immune system, changes in glucose and blood pressure, and vascular changes. These kinds of changes are visible in symptoms that are typically associated with the fight-or-flight response. Some examples include changes in rate of breathing (e.g., increased or decreased breathing), increase in perspiration or body temperature, sensations in the stomach and arms/legs, heart palpitations due to more rapid heart beat, and the release of more sugar into the blood to "prime" the body for the exertion of additional energy.

Many of these psychophysiological processes are activated in response to signals from the amygdala to the autonomic nervous system and the adrenal glands (Hart, Gunnar, & Cicchetti, 1996). In terms of specific clinical samples, researchers have empirically documented the effect of traumatic early care experiences on specific aspects of brain structure, such as the volume of the hippocampus, that part of the brain associated with the capacity to integrate memories into a coherent narrative and sense of self; on serotogenic functioning; and on other structural and functional aspects of brain development, as measured by studies using event-related potential (ERP) measurements (Pollak, Cicchetti, Klorman, & Brumaghim, 1997; Stein, Hanna, Vaerum, & Koverola, 1999).

Some children exposed to early trauma develop a dissociative pattern of coping—an extreme version of the fight-or-flight response—that becomes "engrained" in their neurobiological infrastructure. Perry (1995) described how an overreliance on this coping strategy can help to explain the causal pathway by which a *state* may become more engrained and *trait*-like via its effect on the individual's neurobiology. Because this pattern is a commonly recognized clinical presentation, we explore it further in the following vignette.

Sarah is a 24-year-old medical student described as bright, competent, analytical, and focused. In the process of completing her student internships she is evaluated on a monthly basis by the senior physicians with whom she is working. The majority of her evaluations are positive and strong, yet repeatedly it has been observed that she sometimes seems to "disappear" in that she becomes inexplicably inattentive and "hard to reach."

When Sarah was in the latency phase of development, at age 9, she experienced an episode of sexual abuse while away at summer camp. Her efforts to contact her parents were thwarted by the perpetrator (who happened to be the camp director), who removed Sarah's letters from the mail and refused to deliver her family's letters to her. Although Sarah has incomplete explicit memories of the abuse, she does remember the director coming into the cabin at night and threatening her to "pretend to be asleep or else."

Upon return home from the camp experience, Sarah became inconsolable and was unable to articulate the source of her distress to her parents. She reported experiences characteristic of dissociation, such as feeling that she was "floating above her bed" and that she spent most of her playtime "watching herself" play with other children, rather than enjoying a sense of spontaneous and full involvement. Gradually, her overt expression of distress diminished and she "got used to being one way on the inside and one way on the outside"; feeling almost all of the time that "no one really knew her." As time went on, Sarah's considerable strengths, such as her intelligence, provided other constructive avenues for functioning, and she excelled at school and, on the surface, maintained a series of friendships and family relationships. Her entrance into therapy was precipitated by overwhelming anxiety that was diffused to the point that Sarah had little sense of any trigger. She was aware, however, that there were many "blank spots" in her memory of her childhood and adolescence and that, at times, she would feel "like an outsider" in her own life.

In young children, as with adults, the stress response is an important coping mechanism comprised of psychological, physiological, and behavioral elements (Mangelsdorf, Shapiro, & Marzolf, 1994). Lewis (1992) identified three aspects of the stress response that have important clinical implications for practitioners working with children: threshold, dampening, and reactivation:

Threshold: amount of stressful stimulation necessary to produce a response.

Dampening: the child's ability to stop responding to a stimulus once his or her threshold has been exceeded.

Reactivation: the speed with which the child's stress response can be reelicited after reacting to a stressful stimulus and experiencing a dampening response.

Researchers in the cognitive neurosciences now understand many of the neurobiological mechanisms that underlie various aspects of the stress response. Among the most important findings of this work is that neurobiological changes occur in response to unresolved stress that may render a child vulnerable via (1) an increased sensitivity to future stress and (2) a compromised neurobiological capacity to withstand and regulate negative states of affective arousal (Hofer, 1995; Perry et al., 1995).

In the sections to follow, we focus on three groups of vulnerable dyads: (1) adolescent mothers and the risks associated with their maternal behavior to the developmental well-being of their children; (2) depressed mothers and how symptoms of depression may interfere with important aspects of parenting that, in turn, compromise the child's relational environment; and (3) drug-using mothers and the ways in which substance abuse may comprise fetal development as well as the caregiving environment, creating both direct an indirect pathways by which maternal drug usage may impact child development outcomes.

ADOLESCENT MOTHERS AND THEIR CHILDREN

Adolescent mothers and their children present a unique set of challenges to researchers, clinicians, and policy analysts interested in those issues basic to the health and development of children and families. The developmental vulnerability of adolescent mothers and their children has been carefully documented (Flanagan, McGrath, Meyer, & Garcia-Coll, 1995; Furstenberg, Brooks-Gunn, & Levine, 1990; Osofsky, Eberhart-Wright, Ware, & Hann, 1992; Seitz & Apfel, 1999; Shapiro & Mangelsdorf, 1994; Shapiro, 2003). This multidisciplinary literature has provided insight into the developmental risks, for parent and child, associated with early childbearing and emphasizes adolescent parenting as an important social concern, even as the birth rate among adolescents has continued to decline in recent years.

The focus of studies on adolescent parenting has shifted over time, broadening from a focus on the risks of early parenthood *to the adolescent* to the ways in which early childbearing poses risks not only for young mothers but for their children and extended families as well (Pope et al., 1993). Studies have shown that although substantial variation in the quality of adaptation to early parenthood exists among adolescent mothers, the children of adolescents may be more uniformly at risk for developmental disturbance and delay than children born to older mothers (Shapiro & Mangelsdorf, 1994).

Three sets of literature may be combined to support a focus on the parenting behavior of adolescent mothers as an important factor in the etiology of the developmental delays observed in the children of adolescent mothers. First, a multidisciplinary set of studies has demonstrated the correlation, over time, between parenting behavior, the emerging quality of the parent–child relationship, and a range of social, physical, emotional, and cognitive developmental outcomes in infants and young children (Ainsworth et al., 1978; Schore, 1994; Shapiro & Applegate, 2000; Stern, 1985; Winnicott, 1965d). Increasingly, this literature has reflected a true biopsychosocial perspective as research in the cognitive neurosciences has documented the neurobiological underpinnings and correlates of parent–infant interaction and the nature of early brain development in infants and young children (Schore, 1997). Second, Research has shown significant differences in the parenting behavior of adolescent mothers, as compared to that of adult mothers who are matched on important contextual factors such as marital, educational, and socioeconomic status (Shapiro, 2002; Ward, Botyanski, Plunkett, & Carlson, 1991). Lastly are those studies that describe differentially negative outcomes for children of adolescent mothers as opposed to the developmental trajectories observed in children of older mothers.

Thus, although variation in parenting capacity exists among adolescent mothers, as within any high-risk group, appreciable developmental risk accrues to the children of adolescent mothers due, in part, to relational vulnerability in the adolescent mother–child dyad. Principles of infant mental health are useful in designing interventions that support the adolescent mother–child relationship, promote contingently responsive caregiving, and address the full range of contextual factors affecting the well-being of adolescent mothers and their children.

Parenting Behavior of Adolescent Mothers

An underlying assumption of many process models of parenthood is that to be a parent is to be an adult. Yet adolescent mothers face the tasks and stresses of parenthood in unique social, psychological, economic, and developmental contexts (Garcia-Coll, Hoffman, & Oh, 1987; Shapiro & Mangelsdorf, 1994). As developmentally oriented researchers have long recognized, maturational differences between children and adults must be taken into account in the assessment and interpretation of behavior. Both adaptive and maladaptive behaviors are best understood within a developmental context (Schamess, 1991). However, few studies have empirically examined models of adult parenthood in terms of their utility in predicting patterns of risk and resilience among adolescent mothers. Some of these studies have found that determinants of parenting competence among adolescents are patterned differently than would be predicted by existing models of adult parenting competence (Shapiro & Mangelsdorf, 1994). For example, increased social support (e.g., from the adolescent's mother) may not always be associated with increased parenting competence, as we would expect to find among adult mothers.

Research shows that behavioral differences exist between adolescent and older mothers (Brooks-Gunn, 1990; Chase-Lansdale, Brooks-Gunn, & Paikoff, 1991; Culp, Culp, Osofsky, & Osofsky, 1991; Osofsky et al., 1992). The effect of maternal age on parenting capacity is more pronounced among younger adolescents (Ward & Carlson, 1995; Shapiro & Mangelsdorf, 1994). Younger adolescents are more likely to display less acceptance of the maternal role, less cooperativeness and contingent responsivity, and less sensitivity in their perception of infant cues (Nath, Borkowski, Whitman, & Schellenbach, 1991). The extent to which such group differences are found is mediated by many factors known to shape parenting behavior in both adolescent and adult mothers. These factors include socioeconomic status, marital status, level of educational attainment, psychosocial maturity, psychological health, the presence of negative life events, and the availability of social support. However, the pathways of influence connecting these factors (e.g., social support) and parenting behavior have been shown to differ between adolescent and adult mothers, as well as between younger and older adolescents (Shapiro & Mangesldorf, 1994). Thus adult models of parenting competence may not be entirely descriptive of the experience of adolescent mothers and their children.

As compared to older mothers, adolescent mothers have been characterized as less verbal in their interactions with their children, more controlling, less contingently responsive, and less sensitive (Brooks-Gunn & Furstenberg, 1986; Osofsky, Eberhart-Wright, Ware, & Hann, 1992). In addition, adolescent mothers are often characterized as expecting either "too much too soon" or "too little, too late." Specifically, adolescent mothers are more likely to have unrealistically high expectations of their infants in the sphere of psychomotor development, as might be evidenced by a young mother expecting a newborn infant to hold his or her own bottle. At the same time, adolescent mothers are also more likely to have unrealistically low expectations of their infants in terms of cognitive and linguistic development. For example, the observation that adolescent mothers are more likely to believe that an infant "can't understand" speech may explain why adolescent mothers have been observed to vocalize less to their children. This finding is important because research has shown that the degree of warm, verbal interactions at 6, 13, and 24 months is associated with measures of cognitive and social competence in toddlerhood. Like-wise, an adolescent mother may be more likely to perceive an infant's cry as an indication of being "spoiled," which, in turn, may result in a lower degree of responsivity and emotional availability; two characteristics asso-ciated with many indicators of child well-being (Emde, 1985).

In summary, when maternal expectations of child development and behavior are based on false assumptions regarding normative develop-ment, they are likely to be out of synchrony with the child's capacities. Such dysynchrony can lead to a cycle of inaccurate signal interpretation and subsequent parental response patterns that are not attuned to the child's physical and emotional needs (Stern, 1985). Once such cycles of dissonant interaction begin, the mother's sense of efficacy may be com-promised (Donovan & Leavitt, 1992). Alternatively, when a mother accu-rately "reads" and responds to her infant's cues, she is likely to get positive feedback regarding her maternal competence. This sense of competence is important to all parents but perhaps especially so to very young parents, whose sense of parental role identification is least supported societally and potentially most at risk (Schamess, 1991).

Research on the effects of early parenthood on child development has focused more on a range of cognitive and educational outcomes than on social and emotional development (Carter, Osofsky, & Hann, 1992). How-ever, developmental research highlights the relationship between socioe-motional development and cognitive growth and capacity (Schore, 1994; Shapiro & Applegate, 2000). Thus research that suggests the presence of deficits in cognitive development among children of adolescent mothers also raises important questions about the quality of the caregiving envi-ronment, the influence of a range of contextual factors such as poverty and social isolation, and the ways in which these factors exert develop-mental influence over time.

By elementary school, children of adolescent mothers are more likely to be described as distractible, disorganized, low in frustration tolerance, and impulsive. Such characteristics are often associated with being "un-ready to learn" and with indicators of school failure such as grade reten-tion (Brooks-Gunn & Furstenberg, 1986). However, as Moore and Snyder pointed out, "there is a strong selectivity into adolescent parenthood, and even more so, into school failure" (1990, p. 32). These researchers highlighted the importance of antecedents to early parenthood itself, as well as and other variables such as maternal educational attainment and socioeconomic status that are also associated with cognitive development and academic achievement.

Research on the social and emotional development of children born to adolescent mothers suggests important areas for assessment and intervention in this at-risk population (Ponirakis, Susman, & Stifter, 1999). Some studies have suggested that the children of adolescent mothers are less likely to be securely attached than are children of older mothers (Osofsky et al., 1992). Clinical researchers have observed that adolescent mothers face particular challenges, derived both from normative developmental issues and the presence of other risks such as depression, in the regulation of affect and in sustaining empathic interaction with their children (Osofsky et al., 1992). These findings are particularly important in light of research that described the importance of early caregiving to brain development in early life and, specifically, to the development of the neurobiological substrate of a range of adaptive capacities (Schore, 1994; Shapiro & Applegate, 2000).

Studies of the caregiving context for children of adolescent mothers are complicated because the circle of care provided to the infant often includes the adolescent mother as well as grandparent care or the care of others in the extended family (Radin, Oyserman, & Benn, 1990). The presence of a caring grandparent or other adult caregiver has been shown to buffer young children from some of the risk associated with adolescent parenthood. Still, other research suggests that although the presence of grandparent care may be helpful in the short run, it may challenge the adolescent mother's identification with the maternal role and thus interfere with the process of parent–child attachment (Ward et al., 1991). This conflict is an example of the dual developmental crisis associated with adolescent motherhood. One of the primary social challenges is finding a multigenerational solution that enables the adolescent to continue on an age-appropriate developmental track while, at the same time, providing a developmental context for the young child that potentiates developmental growth and competence.

> Sally is a 15-year-old adolescent mother who attends an alternative high school for adolescent mothers and their children. Her daughter, Alyssa, is 10 months old; while Sally attends class at the high school, Alyssa is cared for in the infant nursery located in the school building. At home, Sally and Alyssa live with Sally's mother who often provides additional care for Alyssa.
>
> Sally was asked by the parent education coordinator at the school to "play with" her daughter the way she usually would at home. This was done to afford the parent educator an opportunity to observe an interaction between Sally and Alyssa that was relatively unstructured and not in a feeding context. Sally and Alyssa sat together on a play mat in a quiet section of the infant nursery. Several toys, including a musical rattle and stacking rings, were available. Sally sat on the mat, motionless and quiet, initiating no interaction with Alyssa. Alyssa, on the other hand, seemed eager to explore the toys and made efforts to crawl toward objects. As she reached the stacking rings, Sally picked them up and moved them to the other side of the play mat, out of Alyssa's reach. When Alyssa reached for the rattle and turned to share a happy expression with Sally, Sally continued to be unresponsive. Slowly, Alyssa's smile faded and subtle signs of anxiety began to emerge. In addition to ceasing her exploration of the toys, Alyssa began to drool and to rock back and forth in a sitting position. When Alyssa heard a school bell ring, she brightened and again looked toward her mother, but when no response was forthcoming, Alyssa soon began to cry, and the observation session was ended.

The Developmental Ecology of Adolescent Parenthood

The study of adolescent parenthood presents an opportunity to observe the superimposition of two developmental phases, adolescence and parenthood, that are usually temporally separated in our society. The developmental tasks of adolescence may conflict with those of parenthood, creating a compromised psychological context for the development of adolescent mothers and their children. It is in this sense that adolescent motherhood may precipitate a "dual developmental crisis" (Sadler & Catrone, 1983). For example, the normative adolescent behavior of experimenting with various roles in the process of identity formation may conflict with the parenting task of fixed maternal role identification (Elkind & Bowen, 1979).

The idea of unresolved developmental conflict in parenthood is not new (Benedek, 1959; Fraiberg, 1980; Lieberman & Pawl, 1990). In many models of adult parenthood, mastery over the developmental tasks of adolescence is understood as a predictor of parenting competence (Fraiberg, 1980). Among adult parents, it is "unresolved adolescent conflicts" which are thought to precipitate some of the most severe parent–child relational problems (Sameroff & Fiese, 1990). When an adolescent mother's own developmental trajectory is interrupted by early or "off-timed" parenthood (Russell, 1980), the development of the adolescent's current and future parenting capacity may be impaired, creating an at-risk relational environment for the developing child.

In her early work on the adolescent experience of pregnancy, Hatcher (1976) noted that the "experience of any adolescent crisis, and especially one of a psychophysiological nature, is influenced by the developmental stage during which it happens to occur" (p. 408). Extending this argument to encompass not only pregnancy, but parenthood as well allows for the construction of hypotheses regarding the influence of normative adolescent development on the psychological experience of early parenthood, and the ways in which the normative tasks of adolescent development may conflict with the developmental tasks associated with parenthood. This view also reflects current understanding in models of developmental psychopathology that suggest that behavior, both functional and dysfunctional, must be understood within the context of normative development.

Mastery over the developmental tasks of adolescence requires the negotiation of stressful life events for all adolescents (Brooks-Gunn, 1990; Dacey & Travers, 2002). Adolescent mothers must negotiate not only normative, age-related developmental transformations, but the early acquisition of the maternal role as well (Kissman & Shapiro, 1990). Moreover, adolescent mothers are more likely to inhabit a social ecology characterized by high levels of stress and low levels of personal, familial, or societal support. Together, these factors are associated with risks to parenting competence and child development outcomes as well.

> Jackie is an 18-year-old mother of a 2-year-old son. Since her child was born, Jackie and her son have continued to live with Jackie's mother and grandmother. This intergenerational family has provided uniquely important support that has enabled Jackie to finish high school. In addition, Jackie's son, Kelly, is clearly securely attached to Jackie's mother and grandmother. As Jackie gets ready to graduate from high school, she is also preparing to enter college and wishes to live independently with her son, apart from her mother and grandmother. This prospective move has raised enormous conflict in the family, primarily because Jackie's mother has been the primary caretaker of Kelly. Although Kelly is attached to Jackie, when he is hurt, scared, or anxious, he first reaches to his grandmother. In addition, his coping behaviors are primarily focused on his grandmother, not his mother, with whom he has had positive, but less consistent, contact. The infant mental health specialist who has been working with Jackie and her family is concerned about how the somewhat normative conflicts around separation/individuation between Jackie and her mother will impact Kelly. The specialist continues to work with Jackie, her mother, and grandmother to find a solution that can support Jackie's growing need for independence and also sustain the important relational ties that Kelly has formed with his extended caregiving circle.

Psychological Issues in The Study of Adolescent Development

Three psychological processes are often the focus of developmental and clinical research on adolescent development: (1) the nature of separation and individuation from one's family of origin, (2) the processes of identity formation, and (3) the emergence of increased cognitive complexity in adolescence. Each of these processes is considered in this section in terms of its import for parenting capacity and revisited in the following section on the subphases of adolescent development.

SEPARATION AND INDIVIDUATION

By naming adolescence the "second phase of separation and individuation," Blos (1967) drew a parallel between a primary developmental task of adolescence and the first phase of separation/individuation that occurs at, or around, the end of the second year of life. In both phases there is a maturational push toward higher levels of autonomous functioning that requires (1) continued psychological change with regard to primary relationships, (2) adaptation to increased maturational demands, and (3) temporary vulnerability, as tasks once shared between child and caregiver are performed with increasing autonomy and require the integration of new capacities and coping skills.

Historically, psychoanalytic theorists have viewed the processes of separation and individuation as being intricately tied to the process of ego identity development (Hatcher, 1976; Kroger, 2000). The process of ego identity development requires the adolescent to synthesize past identifications with current experience and maturational demands. Adequate progress in the processes of separation and individuation results, by the end of adolescence, in important structural changes in personality. Self and object representations acquire internal stability, no longer as dependent on external sources of validation, lending a constancy to self-esteem and the internal regulation of affective states. When adequate gains toward separation and individuation do not occur, ego functions that normally become solidified in adolescence, such as reality testing and the regulation of self-esteem, may remain overly dependent on external sources and thus prone to regression under stress. More recently, other theorists have discussed how multiple pathways toward identity development are possible (Kroger, 2000). In particular, the ability to form identity *via* involvement in relationships is an important consideration. For adolescent mothers, this may be uniquely important as they continue their own development in the context of the relational demands of parenting (Josselson, 1987).

The developmental demands and social realities of parenthood may conflict with the tasks of separation and individuation (Ward et al., 1991).

Normatively, increasing autonomy and reducing dependency are salient aspects of adolescent development. However, the acquisition of the maternal role often heightens the adolescent's dependency on her family of origin. If this upsurge in dependency occurs in a psychological context in which the adolescent had hoped that becoming a mother would "make me an adult" or "get me out from under" parental rules and authority, the dissonance between expectation and reality may precipitate feelings of disappointment, depression, or resentment. These feelings may be directed toward the adolescent's parent, herself, or more unhappily, toward the developing infant. In these cases, resolving the adolescent's dependency conflicts in a way that promotes adaptation for both the adolescent and her child may require a multigenerational solution. The adolescent's own parent(s) may need support in understanding the adolescent's simultaneous need for, and rejection of, his or her assistance. Similarly, the adolescent may need assistance in coping with the continuous dependency needs of her own child. Thus the impact of early parenthood on the adolescent processes of separation and individuation is shaped by (1) where in the adolescent process parenthood occurs, (2) how well prepared the adolescent was, prior to parenthood, to engage these tasks of adolescence, and (3) the capacity of the adolescent's family to provide a nurturant environment that is sensitive to the developmental needs of both the adolescent and her child.

EGO IDENTITY

Ego identity development in adolescence focuses on tasks inherent to the internalization of an adult personality structure (Erikson, 1958; Josselson, 1987; Cote & Levine, 1988). The process of ego identity formation in adolescence require a reorientation of interpersonal relationships (e.g., the relationship between child and parent), an expanded view of possible roles for the self (Nurius & Markus, 1991), and the consolidation of emerging ego strengths.

Ego identity refers to specific characteristics of personality structure that are construed as either ego strengths or deficits, and which are manifested in functions such as: (1) organization of affective expression, (2) capacity for impulse control, (3) cognitive complexity, (4) quality of defensive structures, and (5) the capacity for relationship and work commitments. Ego identity refers not only to "who one is" but to "how one feels about one's self" and to "what one does" (Josselson, 1987).

Erikson (1958) viewed identity development as a lifelong process. However, because of the depth and breadth of the cognitive, social, psychological, and physical changes that occur during adolescence, this life phase was deemed the "identity stage" of development in Erikson's model. A primary assumption in this model of identity development is the idea that separation and individuation are important precursors to identity attainment. Several theorists have suggested that the focus on individuation as a precursor to the capacity for intimacy may be more descriptive of the "traditional" male experience in our society and that it devalues the traditionally "female" characteristics of affiliation and cooperativeness (Kroger, 2000). Other empirical investigations of identity development in adolescence have begun to go beyond the traditional components of identity to reflect the importance of domains such as relational experience and commitments—constructs clearly relevant to our understanding of parenthood (Grotevant & Cooper, 1982).

As with the processes of separation and individuation, when parenthood occurs during adolescence the process of ego identity development may be disrupted (Ward et al., 1991). Although adolescents are able to become parents without engaging in emotionally intimate relationships, the tasks of parenting require a consistently high level of intimate engagement. And, whereas the normative tasks of identity development during adolescence often include the "trying on and taking off" of various social roles, the successful adaptation to motherhood requires a strong commitment to a particular social role (Shapiro, 2002). Thus it is important to understand not only how the adolescent's level of identity development affects current parenting capacity, but also how the tasks of parenthood may influence ongoing identity development and thus future parenting capacity.

COGNITIVE DEVELOPMENT

Many of the gains associated with cognitive development during adolescence are relevant to aspects of parenting capacity. The attainment of formal operational thought expands the individual's capacity to think abstractly, to self-reflect, and to consider the impact of current behavior on future outcomes. The related capacities to see oneself as others might, to see one's own role in relationship to particular situations, and to accurately conceptualize one's relationships to other people permit the adolescent a greater degree of insight and more accurate judgment (Miller, Miceli, Whitman, & Borkowski, 1996).

Another hallmark of cognitive development during adolescence is the emergence, then diminution, of "adolescent egocentrism" (Elkind & Bowen, 1979). Early and middle adolescence is often characterized as "egocentric"; these adolescents believe that other people are as focused on their ideas and appearance as they are themselves. Elkind and Bowen (1979) referred to this phenomenon as the "imaginary audience." Over time, as adolescents invest more psychological energy into other relationships and external foci, the imaginary audience lessens and they are better able to relate to others as separate individuals with needs and concerns of their own.

Adolescents who become mothers while still maintaining a high level of egocentrism may be unable to accurately perceive or respond to a child's intentions or needs. A baby may continue to be seen as more of a reflection of the adolescent's own needs than as a separate person with reality-based needs of his or her own. For example, an adolescent mother who sees her 3-month-old crying may say, "She's just mad because we're still at school." This statement, clearly a misperception of an infant's cry signal, is a product of the young adolescent's inability to take the perspective of the child.

All parents learn how to parent by trial and error, learning from mistakes and abstracting from such experiences in ways that remediate their future actions (Whitman, Borkowski, Schellenbach, & Nath, 1987). Adolescent mothers may be limited in their learning capacity by concrete operational thinking, which does not include the ability to abstract from present to future experiences. The idea that adolescent mothers may be more concrete in how they conceptualize parenting also has implications for the development of interventions. Many parent education programs are designed to teach parents about child developmental milestones; such teaching is abstract. Interventions designed for adolescents must be primarily present focused and concrete in nature.

In summary, the cognitive immaturity of adolescent mothers may contribute to deficits in parenting competence. Adolescent egocentrism and concrete operational thinking may interfere with the development of empathic parenting behavior. These normative developmental indices of adolescence may contribute to adolescent maternal behavior that is sometimes found to be less empathic, less contingently responsive, and less appropriate than the behavior of adult mothers.

MATERNAL DEPRESSION

Numerous studies and clinical reports have highlighted the developmental vulnerability of children whose parents have untreated affective disorders such as major depression. During infancy and the early years, developmental well-being is critically tied to the emotional stability and availability of the child's primary caregivers (Cohn & Tronick, 1989). Children of depressed mothers have higher rates of many developmental deficits, including problems with the regulation of behavior and attention, higher rates of conduct disorder and separation anxiety, and, higher rates of childhood depression (Dawson, Frey, & Panagiotides, 1997). Longitudinally, children of depressed mothers also have been observed to have more insecure attachments, less developed social skills, and more problematic peer relationships (Campbell, Cohn, & Neyers, 1995; Field et al., 1996; Dawson, Frey, Self, Panagiotides, Hessl, Yamada, & Rinaldi, 1999).

Because the early years of life represent a sensitive period with regard to those aspects of child development most germane to the regulation of emotion and affect, young children are uniquely vulnerable to the effects of maternal depression. Research has shown that sustained periods of maternal affective disorders, especially when they occur early in a baby's life, create more developmental disruption and risk (Schore, 2000). Thus primary prevention of maternal depression as well as prompt assessment and intervention of existing cases of maternal depression are important foci of programs designed to support the well-being of children.

As has been reviewed elsewhere in this volume, the parenting behavior of the child's primary caregiver comprises the primary developmental context of infancy and early childhood. To the extent that maternal depression alters the relational environment of the infant and young child, it is understood to be related to the development of attachment quality and the many related indices of developmental well-being. Research on the impact of depression on maternal behavior has shown that depressed mothers exhibit lower maternal responsivity and sensitivity, are less emotionally available, display more negative mood states, and are less able to provide auxiliary support to the child's emerging attempts at affect regulation (Tronick & Weinberg, 1998). Several additional ways in which the parenting behavior of depressed mothers differs from those who are not depressed include slowness to respond to the infant's bids for interaction, negative or critical verbal comments directed toward or about the infant, difficulty in setting limits on the child's behavior, and less provision of appropriate stimulation (Field, 1995). Recent studies (Dawson et al., 1992) have shown that, within a group of dyads whose mothers had scored high on depression, the mothers demonstrated less positive gaze and positive touch and the infants scored lower on "positive face" displays and higher on "head aversion." In infancy, behaviors such as gaze aversion represent one of the few motoric capacities that infants can draw upon to "shut out" or withdraw from psychologically painful and nonsupporting parent–infant interactions (Dawson, Grofer-Klinger, Panagiotides, Hilld, Spieker, & Frey, 1992).

Maternal depression is a serious risk factor that manifests in a variety of ways. From the standpoint of prevention and treatment, it is important that clinicians be aware of how a particular individual might manifest depression, and the specific ways in which the symptomatology of depression impacts each parent–child dyad. Research has shown that for some depressed mothers, parenting behavior is characterized by a lack of interaction and responsivity to the infant's needs and bids for attention (Field, 1995; Field, Estroff, Tando, del Valle, Malphurs, & Hart, 1996; Lundy, Field, Pickens, & Cigales, 1997; Lyons-Ruth, Bronfman, & Parsons, 1999). In other parent–child dyads, maternal depression can become manifest as overintrusiveness and overstimulation, similarly disregarding of the infant's signals, but in the opposite direction (Meritesacker, Bade, Haverkock, & Pauli-Pott, 2004).

Primary developmental goals of infancy and early childhood involve learning, in the context of important attachment relationships, (1) how to identify one's own feelings, (2) how to identify the feelings of others, (3) how to acquire the capacity to regulate affect sufficiently to maintain homeostasis, and (4) how to invest in the object world of people and exploration. Children of depressed mothers are less likely to receive the empathically attuned and contingently responsive care that would contribute to their ability to understand cause-and-effect relationships; most saliently, the relationship between their own internal states and the development of language to describe affective experience. Research has shown that children of depressed mothers, particularly those whose mothers were depressed during the child's infancy and early childhood, are more likely to vigilantly observe their mothers' mood states and to be highly sensitive to relatively small changes in those states (Cicchetti, Rogosch, & Toth, 1998). Even though maternal mood may be responsive to the advent of treatment, the child's early learning environment regarding the nature and regulation of affect may have resulted in styles of interaction, or attachment, and affect regulation that persist beyond the initial alleviation of the parental depression. Certainly, research on brain development in early life has highlighted the finding that the affectively charged relational environment of infancy is closely tied to those aspects of brain development that are primarily responsible for the experience and regulation of affect (Schore, 1994).

The first years of life are understood to be a critical period with regard to the development of the frontal region of the brain. The frontal lobes of the human brain are closely linked to emotional expression and regulation. The left frontal region is generally associated with the expression and regulation of more positive affective states, whereas the right frontal region is associated with less positive emotions such as sadness (Davidson, Ekman, Saron, & Senulis, 1990). Empirical research with infants of depressed mothers has shown more neural activity in the left frontal region than in the right frontal region (Dawson, Frey, Panagiotides, Osterling, & Hessl, 1997). Dawson et al. stated the following:

When the social environment involves a depressed mother, it is possible that the young child experiences negative emotions and poorly regulates states of arousal more frequently and intensely, and that this results in selective amplification of those neural circuits involved in such emotions and arousal regulation mechanisms. . . . Specifically, frequent and repeated interactions between the parent and infant involving displays of negative emotions may serve to selectively amplify specific neuronal circuits involved in negative affect, while failing to amplify neuronal circuits involved in positive affect. (1991, p. 591)

Infants of depressed mothers have been found to exhibit physiological signs of stress such as increased heart rate and higher salivary and cortical levels. In one study, preschool children with chronic exposure to maternal depression showed a greater tendency to focus on negative emotions and thoughts and a greater sensitivity to the negative emotions of others (Dawson, Hessel, & Frey, 1994). As with any relationally vulnerable dyad, an important question becomes how maternal depression may alter the caregiving context in ways that, in turn, affect early brain development and lead to long-lasting effects in terms of child outcomes (Field, 1995; Field, Estroff, Yando, del Valle, Malphurs, & Hart, 1996).

Infants and young children are uniquely dependent on primary caregivers for a relational environment that augments positive feelings of warmth, security, and joy, and mediates against prolonged states of negative affective arousal (e.g., sadness, anxiety). Children of depressed mothers may come to be at risk, in part, because the depressed caregiver may either show a flatness of affect or a disproportionate amount of negative affect. In either case, the caregiver may be emotionally unavailable and unable to respond contingently to the infant's cues. Moreover, a depressed caregiver is less likely to engage in shared states of positive affect, thereby providing less opportunity for the infant's brain to be engaged in a manner that supports the development of positively charged or positively wired connections. This theory relates to the "use-dependency" or "experientially dependent" concept in early brain development in which those synapses that are "fired" more often become more firmly "wired" into the neural architecture of the child's brain.

To the extent that chronic maternal depression is associated with neglect, it is also important to address research on the ways in which early maternal neglect affects the developing child. In animal studies, researchers have shown that early maternal neglect alters the developmental trajectory of the dopamine system (Gunnar, 2001). Disruption of the dopamine system in the brain has been linked to a wide range of disorders in people, including major affective disorders, such as depression, and the susceptibility to substance abuse—disorders which, in turn, create conditions of risk for children parented by individuals suffering with these problematic conditions. Other researchers have shown that a lack of stimulation and interaction, as might be typical in cases of neglect, is associated with some of the most noticeable developmental/behavioral problems in children, such as difficulties with impulse control (Gunnar, 2001; Gunnar, Bruce, & Grotevant, 2000).

Case Example: The Intersection of Depression and Misread Interaction

Frankie is a 4-month-old infant, born full term into an economically struggling family. Frankie's mother and father immigrated to the United States several years ago and have been struggling to make ends meet by doing domestic work for several families. Although Frankie was born full term, he appears not only small for his age but also more lethargic than would be expected of a 4-month-old infant. A medical workup found no physical cause for Frankie's apparent listlessness and lack of interest in people or visual stimuli presented to him during play. Frankie's mother, who herself has little energy and makes very few verbal comments, mentioned that when Frankie is "nosy" (e.g., when he looks around in a new setting), she tells him to "stop being so nosy." She reported that Frankie is a "good baby" because often, when in his crib during the day, he will lie awake and "not bother me for 3 or 4 hours" until he "gets hungry." She also reported that she "doesn't like

the way he's getting fat" and even though the pediatrician has recom-
mended that he start infant cereal, she "doesn't think he needs it."
When Frankie easily cuddled into the arms of the infant observer,
Frankie's mother remarked "See, I don't really make a difference to him
anyway, he doesn't even notice if I'm around."

This case vignette of Frankie describes a pattern of maternal depression in which the mother, although involved with her infant, has little
energy for interaction. Research on early brain development has described the importance of affectively attuned, positively charged verbal
interactions that help the developing child to augment positive experience and cope with negative states of affective arousal (Gunnar, 2001).
In addition, this research highlights the ways in which such patterns of
interaction are key to the development of those systems involved in the
regulation of affect and attention, and in the development of language
that, over time, can be used by the child to represent and mediate internal states of mind and experiences (Siegel, 1999). In Frankie's case, his
mother misinterprets Frankie's passivity as a sign of being a "good baby."
An alternative hypothesis is that Frankie may have come to experience
interactions with his mother as unsatisfying and, perhaps, even anxiety
producing; instead he opts to withdraw into himself at a critical developmental phase in which interaction with primary caregivers is a key avenue of growth and development. Frankie's mother also misinterprets
her son's natural curiosity as "nosiness" and does not reinforce it, because she does not make positive attributions about Frankie's interest in
the external world. Her low self-esteem, often associated with depression, is evident in her attributions, or thinking, about the ways in which
Frankie responds to other people as well. To the extent that Frankie is
able to be soothed by others, his mother feels personally rejected — as
opposed to viewing his ability to respond as a positive characteristic of
son that is perhaps related to a positive relational environment. Overall,
Frankie's case shows how cycles of misread and misunderstood interactions between infant and caregiver can be related to patterns of depressive symptoms and pose risks to the development of secure attachment

and to those aspects of early social–emotional development related to early interactive experience.

Case Example: Maternal Depression and Infant Vigilance

Claire is a healthy 11-month-old infant of a depressed mother. Born physically and neurologically intact, Claire moved through the first half of her first year of life with no apparent delays or complications. During the last several months, however, Claire's parents have been entrenched in marital conflict over the presence of Claire's father's daughter from a previous marriage. Claire's mother's affect and mood have steadily deteriorated, as has the consistency with which she empathically responds to Claire's bids for attention and interaction. Claire's mother shows intermittent and highly negative facial expressions that, seen from Claire's perspective, must seem to "come over" her mother. Steadily, Claire has begun to focus less of her attention on exploring her toys and enjoying positively charged interactions. Instead, she vigilantly attends to her mother's facial expressions, searching for a "clue" about her mother's affective state. Rather than the social referencing we would expect to see of an infant at this age, wherein the infant "looks back" to mother in an effort to share excitement or for guidance as to whether a particular action (e.g., going up the stairs) is safe or not, Claire seems to have gotten increasingly still, and she focuses primarily on searching her mother's face. When Claire observes her mother's facial expressions becoming more negative, Claire begins to show signs of anxiety (e.g., drooling, anticipatory crying, unable to sustain focus on play) and, if not quickly soothed, her distress escalates to a dysregulated state of crying. Claire is relatively unable to self-soothe or to easily receive soothing from others.

The case of Claire shows a different pattern of maternal depressive symptomatology and how it may manifest in the mother–child interaction by impacting the developing infant's capacity for affect regulation. Claire, a healthy 11-month-old, already shows a pattern descriptive of children whose caregivers have affective disorders. Claire's vigilance in monitoring her mother's mood states, including her search for facial clues of any changes, can be seen as an early coping strategy on Claire's part; an effort to create predictability where much lability exists. It is likely that no one else in Claire's immediate environment is as sensitive to these microaffective changes as is Claire. To Claire, changes in her mother's facial expression have come to represent loss; loss of the emotionally available caregiving figure. In addition, changes in her mother's mood state also signal anxiety to Claire because they serve as a prelude, or forecast, of what may be coming. Because Claire is only 11 months old, she is limited as to her repertoire of self-soothing behaviors in the face of this potential loss and anxiety. What an observer is likely to see is an infant who may turn away from her natural state of exploration and connection, becoming more dysregulated, as evidenced by body discomfort, an increase in drooling, a lack of muscle tone, or efforts at self-soothing, such as non-nutritive sucking, twirling of hair, stillness, or lack of interest in play.

The case of Claire is highly relevant to the discussion of the applied value of research on brain development in early life. In Claire's case, we can see that her mother's depressive stance creates challenge for her, not only in the regulation of her own affective states, but additionally in the ways in which her need to self-soothe and cope with anxiety may hinder her opportunities for learning in other ways, such as the exploration of the object world through play and spontaneous social interaction. To the extent that Claire has become preoccupied with monitoring her mother's affective state, she is spending less of her energy on coming to understand her *own* internal experience and likely does not have access to a caregiving figure that is reflecting back to her important data about her own experience. Thus, Claire's relational environment does not provide her with a mirror, through either maternal facial expression or language, of her own internal world. As Claire has become more attuned to changes in her mother's expression of affect, she has also become more anxious about the meaning of these changes, because they have come to be associated with loss of maternal availability.

Each of these elements is, in turn, related to important indices of those aspects of early brain development related to affective and cognitive functioning.

Case Example:
Maternal Depression and Forced Infant Independence

Roberta is a 27-year-old mother of two young children. Economically stressed and living in unsatisfactory housing, Roberta has had few sources of consistent support in her role of mother. Roberta's youngest child, Anthony, is 14 months old and appears to be extremely independent for his age. As Roberta sits in the living room with the television on, her attention does not seem focused, and she does not respond to household noises and signals as they occur. For example, if the phone rings she is likely not to answer it, and if she hears a child's cry in the other room, she is unlikely to respond. Anthony, able to walk, wanders through the apartment by himself. Even as he sits down near his mother to play, he seems to be very much "alone." Observation of Anthony shows that he rarely, if at all, looks to his mother in a "social referencing" manner to share affect or to gain reassurance or support in his exploration of the environment. When Anthony falls in the context of play and cries in pain, Roberta exclaims, "Why do you always have to get into so much trouble," and offers no reassurance or empathic support. Slowly, Anthony stops crying but is so exhausted from his independent play and need to self-soothe that he falls asleep on the living room floor, withdrawing from efforts to interact with his mother and from his exploratory activities.

This dyad provides an example of how maternal emotional unavailability can create affective pain for a young child. For Anthony, normative signals do not correspond to maternal efforts and response. Over time, Anthony has learned to signal for his mother less, withdrawing in an effort to self-soothe. Anthony's young age places him at risk for negative outcome because he cannot rely on auxiliary support from his mother.

DRUG USAGE AND PARENTING

The impact of parental drug usage on fetal, infant, and child development has been widely studied (Chasnoff, Anson, Hatcher, Stenson, & Iaukea, 1998). Although debate exists as to the short- and long-term consequences to the child of prenatal maternal drug use, some harmful effects are generally recognized. Even though not all illicit substances result in children being born addicted, many other deleterious effects are associated with prenatal exposure to drugs such as alcohol, cocaine, marijuana, heroin, methadone, amphetamines, and PCP. Complications include premature birth, low birth weight, smaller head circumference, premature separation of the placenta from the womb, and insufficient access to oxygen. Some problems evident at birth diminish as times goes on, but other, subtler problems in mental, emotional, and neurological functioning may persist over time (Tronick & Beeghly, 1992).

Children born to substance-abusing parents are considered to be at "developmental risk" in a number of ways. Early research on the impact of drug abuse on child development focused primarily on the impact of prenatal exposure to a variety of drugs. From the perspective of how drug usage impacts the caregiving environment, two interrelated issues emerge. First, children born addicted to illicit substances face a range of physical and developmental challenges in recovery and present complex caregiving demands for primary caregivers. These children tend to be, among other things, easily agitated and aroused, have difficulty achieving state regulation, and may be difficult to soothe (Shapiro et al., 2001). At the same time, if children are being cared for by parents actively involved in addiction or substance abuse, the caregiving environment is likely to be less than optimal, characterized by inadequate caregiving ranging from neglect to abuse.

The effects of parental drug usage on infant and child development present complex research questions. It is important to assess the direct impact of a particular drug, for example, on the developing fetus, as well as the impact of a particular drug, or drugs, on aspects of parental perception, decision making and behavior, which will, in turn, also affect child development outcomes (Carter & Larson, 1997). Much work has been done on identifying the impact of many biological insults including prenatal exposure to neurotoxins, on the developing brain. As was pointed out by the National Research Council publication, "From Neurons to Neighborhoods" (Shonkoff & Phillips, 2000), prenatal and early life brain development are highly "plastic" and thus sensitive to the advent of neurotoxins and deleterious experience. At the same time, this plasticity affords an important focus for preventive intervention, because altered situational circumstance can also have a positive effect on early brain development.

Among those factors identified as commonly presenting a risk to prenatal development are exposure to alcohol, lead, tobacco, and cocaine. Researchers have pointed out that a simplistic view of exposure has less clinical meaning than a perspective that takes into account the timing of exposure (e.g., when in gestation the exposure occurred), the amount/ dose of the exposure (e.g., how much of the substance was the developing fetus exposed to?), and the chronicity of the exposure (e.g., over what period of time did the exposure occur?). Other factors have also been identified as posing risks to early brain development, including chronic stress, lack of access to prenatal care or health care, exposure to untreated infection, and malnutrition (Chasnoff, Anson, Hatcher, Stenson, Iaukea, & Randolph, 1998).

The impact of parental drug usage on any particular outcome, such as prenatal and early brain development, must be understood in a truly biopsychosocial context that considers multiple risk factors as potentially additive and most certainly as recursively interactive (Chasnott, Anson, Hatcher, Stenson, & Iaukea, 1998). In addition to the parental drug use itself, deleterious effects on the developing child may also be associated with those conditions that precipitated parental drug use (e.g., parental depression, inability to self-soothe, chronic stress) or to conditions that exist as a consequence of parental drug usage (e.g., parental inattention and neglect, lack of access to adequate financial resources, lack of access to adequate health care and food, and the inability of some parents to navigate the service delivery system successfully).

A summary prepared by the National Clearinghouse on Child Abuse and Neglect (1993; NCCAN) highlights the ways in which the use of illicit drugs can profoundly affect parenting behavior and, in turn, a range of child development outcomes. Several of these areas are related, either directly or indirectly, to the development of secure attachment relationships. These include:

1. *Parental access to sufficient income for providing for the child's basic needs and stability, including access to shelter, nutrition, medical care, child care, and education.* For parents with an active addiction, it is likely that the financial resources of the family will be strained by the cost of the addiction itself, or that the addiction will interfere with the stability of other important resources such as housing and nutrition.

2. *The importance of parental capacity for nurturance, sensitivity, and empathic relatedness.* In the parent–child relationship, the responsibility for nurturance, sensitivity, and empathic responsivity lies with the adult caregiving figure(s). If a parent is involved in illicit drug usage, his or her ability to correctly perceive and respond to the needs of the infant may be limited. This limitation is particularly problematic if the infant was born, secondary to prenatal drug exposure, with unusual or challenging caregiving needs.

3. *The provision of external structure.* In infancy and early childhood, children rely almost solely upon adults for the provision of a home environment that is characterized by sufficient structure, healthfulness, and predictability. In combination with access to nurturance, this kind of external structure helps the developing child to begin to form an internalized sense of structure. In a family under severe stress, be it economic or related to parental drug usage, it may be less likely that the child's living situation will be sufficiently safe and sanitary. Young children, eager to explore, need protection from unsafe substances, hot stoves, and myriad other safety concerns. In addition, children in substance-abusing families are more likely to be given age-inappropriate responsibilities for younger siblings, creating risk for both younger and older children.

Case Example: A Mother in Recovery from Addiction

Melanie is a 25-year-old mother of three who is in recovery from her addictions to heroin and cocaine. While in her phase of active addiction,

Melanie's three children (ages 2, 3, and 5) were cared for by a foster family. Prior to the children's placement in foster care, they experienced considerable instability in their mother's care. Melanie would often leave the three children alone as she went out in search of drugs. When the children were left alone, they had little ability to care for themselves; on one occasion, they were found foraging for food in a neighbor's trash can. The children showed very little emotion and evidenced almost no expectation that adults would be responsive to them or sources of comfort or shared positive affect. Closely attached to each other, the children evidence signs of panic and anxiety if efforts are made to separate them, even for brief periods of time.

Melanie now expresses frustration that the "children don't seem to trust" her and "prefer each other" to her. While continuing to make efforts at her recovery, Melanie often talks about feeling that her children should "appreciate" more of what she is trying to do on her own behalf and that they are somewhat "spoiled" compared to the way that she herself grew up. More than once, Melanie has stated that her childhood experiences were "good enough" for her and that even though she "never got any attention," she "turned out fine." From this perspective, Melanie often wonders, "If it was good enough for me, why isn't it good enough for them, too?"

The above vignette highlights some important problems in working with children of drug-addicted parents. Melanie's drug addiction, while certainly multiply determined, may have begun as an effort to self-soothe and protect against affects that were too overwhelming or painful. Although an outside observer of Melanie's childhood would recognize that Melanie experienced substantial neglect and sometimes abuse, she herself only describes "being alone." On a conscious, or verbal, level Melanie does not express a belief that she was neglected. In addition, although she is able to describe memories of being left alone, without access to adult support, she does not seem to experience affect associated with these memories. Clinical research in infant mental health has shown that in order for a parent to have empathy with the emotional pain of their children, the parent must be able to have empathy for his or her own childhood experiences. Melanie may be unable to identify or empathize with her children's emotions because she herself may have been too overwhelmed as a child, too far into "survival mode," to let herself feel the affect associated with her own experiences. An infant mental health approach would focus on encouraging Melanie's ability to understand her children's feelings via building a relationship with Melanie that also focuses on offering empathy *to Melanie*. She may also need assistance in recognizing that what she perceives as "rejection" by her children may be related to their own fears of loss in relationship to their mother. Rather than seeing her children's behavior as a disinterest in her, she may be helped to see it as uncertainty as to her emotional availability to them.

The primary goal of this chapter was to describe the vulnerability of those parent–child dyads whose relational stability is threatened by developmental, social, environmental, or psychological factors. Research in the cognitive neurosciences certainly highlights the importance of early care experiences to brain development in early life. This research is an important complement to our psychosocial understanding of early attachment and its effects on developmental well-being. From a social work perspective, research on the neurobiological effects of early relational care is critical to our ability to delineate the processes by which developmental risk is accrued by children in at-risk care environments. In addition, we have learned that during the first years of life, neurobiological patterns are formed that, although plastic to some degree, are also significantly enduring—which may explain why at-risk children tend to retain an internal fragility and vulnerability even when the external, situational context has been altered and improved.

Chapter 7

INFANT MENTAL HEALTH

From Understanding to Prevention

MANY ASPECTS OF BRAIN development in early life are related to infant and child mental health. As noted throughout this volume, the early years of life comprise a sensitive period with regard to those aspects of development that are central to the capacities to experience, express, and regulate affect. The neurobiological substrate of these capacities forms in the context of early caregiving relationships and is carried forward into latency, adolescence, and beyond.

For clinicians working with vulnerable children and families, the emphasis on the importance of early experience presents both challenge and hope. On the one hand, recognition that the quality of care a child receives in the first years of life is an important protective factor highlights the vulnerability of those children who lack consistent access to stable and empathic care. As social workers, we are all too familiar with the many groups of at-risk children whose early life experiences are characterized by disruption, chaos, neglect, and deprivation. On the other hand, knowledge of the plasticity of early brain development and the specific mechanisms by which early experience shapes postnatal brain development

119

highlights the potential for early *prevention* and reinforces the need for *interventions* with at-risk children and their families.

Infant mental health is a multidisciplinary field of clinical work, research, policy development, and advocacy that has as its primary goal the promotion of healthy and strong early caregiving relationships that can support the health and development of infants, young children, and their families. From a clinical perspective, the field of infant mental health is broadly focused on the ways in which infants and young children experience, express, and regulate affect and the importance of secure attachment to the developing child's capacity to explore the environment and to engage in learning (Lieberman & Zeanah, 1995; Lieberman, Wieder, & Fenichel, 1997). From an infant mental health perspective the definition of "who the client is" includes the child in the context of the family, focusing not on the importance of a particular family structure but on the availability of the kind of sensitive, empathically attuned, and consistent care shown to be facilitative of optimal social and emotional development in infancy and early childhood.

From a social work perspective, many of the concepts associated with the field of infant mental health also support a strengths-oriented perspective with children and families; a perspective that values diversity in terms of developmental pathways *and* in terms of how cultural experience shapes family life and child development. In addition, a cornerstone of infant mental health is an emphasis on relationships. The relationship between infants and their primary caregivers is the main focus of assessment, prevention, and intervention in an infant mental health framework. In addition, the relationships between social worker and parent, between social worker and child, and between the parent–child dyad and social service agencies are important foci as well. Thus the beliefs, skills, and interventional methods associated with infant mental health reflect longstanding commitments to children and families within the social work profession.

A review of the basic concepts and methods associated with infant mental health is relevant to our work here, because many children with whom social workers come into contact are at risk due to lack of access to the kinds of consistent and stable care associated with psychological well-being and with optimal brain development in early life. Much of the focus on brain development in early life has centered on the impact of early experience and stimulation on indices of cognitive development and school readiness (Shonkoff & Phillips, 2000). Other researchers have begun to articulate the importance of early experience not only to cognitive development, but to many aspects of social and emotional development that, in turn, support the capacity for effective learning (Siegel, 1999). The concept of *emotional intelligence* (Goleman, 1995) can be used to describe the relationship between affect and cognition and highlights how those aspects of early experience that support the neurobiological substrate of affect regulation are relevant to multiple aspects of intelligence. This concept is relevant to our discussion of infant mental health because "school readiness" relates to each child's early experience, capacity to cope with feelings, and ability to engage in constructive relationships. It is important that clinicians become adept at recognizing the ways in which a lack of access to consistent and empathic care may interfere with the emotional intelligence a child needs to succeed in school.

According to Goleman (1995) emotional intelligence refers to a set of characteristics that includes (1) self-awareness of feelings and emotions; (2) the capacity to regulate states of affect and guide patterns of behavioral responses to affect; (3) self-motivation and the ability to experience, sustain, and direct curiosity; (4) empathy and the capacity to recognize and respond to feelings in other people, perceiving both verbal and nonverbal cues, and (5) using these skills to negotiate interpersonal relationships, over time, by developing capacities for communication, cooperation, impulse control, and frustration tolerance.

Children whose early circle of care is fragmented, chaotic, and bereft of understanding of their emotional needs may lack the opportunity to develop the basic infrastructure of emotional intelligence that is necessary to enable them to fulfill their potential as they move beyond the boundary of the family and into the world of peers and school-based learning. Thus, when we talk about "infant mental health," we have in mind a facilitation of the social and emotional development of children, in the context of caregiving relationships, which, in turn, supports children's emerging capacity to regulate affect sufficiently to sustain investment in the world of family, friendships, and school.

CORE PRINCIPLES OF INFANT MENTAL HEALTH

The infant mental health movement began in the early 1970s as research on the neurological, social, physical, and cognitive competencies of infants was rapidly accumulating. Research on attachment in infancy focused attention on the primacy of early caregiving relationships and the processes by which the *quality* of these relationships shaped important developmental outcomes. Infant mental health, a field pioneered by Selma Fraiberg and her colleagues at the Child Development Project (Fraiberg, Adelson, & Shapiro, 1975), emerged as an innovative way to apply this new knowledge of development to the processes of assessment, prevention, and intervention. Psychodynamically informed, the field of infant mental health raised important questions about the emotional life of infants and young children, and how the emergence of behavioral problems in childhood reflected unresolved emotional conflicts. Yet the field of infant mental health added a new perspective by focusing not only on the internal world of the child but on the internal world of the *caregivers* as an important mediator of parental behavior; a characteristic that, in turn, affects child development itself. In addition, infant mental health spear-headed an important shift in clinical work with young children and their families, in that the strategies were comprehensive in nature, focusing not only on the psychological state of the parent–child relationship but on the family's need for assistance with concrete services, emotional support, and developmental guidance (Weatherston, 2000).

The application of theory and research to practice is an important element of infant mental health. The kinds of research reviewed in this volume are highly relevant to our understanding of social and emotional development in infancy and the ways in which the psychological health of the parent provides an important developmental context for the child, shaping the relational environment in which attachments develop and, relatedly, shaping brain development in early life. As has been reviewed in previous chapters, early brain development is best supported by access to adequate nutrition, freedom from abuse and neglect, and access to stable and consistent care characterized as contingently responsive and infused with an understanding of the infant's internal experience and needs. Moreover, research shows that an important role of caregivers is to minimize the infant's exposure to stress and augment the experiences of positive affect. McKewen (2001) articulated the concept of the "allostatic load," the ways in which unresolved stress creates systemic strain for the developing child, including short- and long-term impact on various brain systems. It is important that babies and young children live in environments that contain a minimal number of stressors and that adult caregivers have a realistic assessment of what kinds of stimuli cause stress for children at different ages. For example, very young infants may experience unpredictability as extremely stressful, much as other infants might find excess noise overwhelming to their immature nervous systems.

Lieberman, Weider and Fenichel (1997) summarized the following basic principles of infant mental health:

1. Even very young infants are understood as "social beings."
2. Individual differences are important to understand.
3. A range of environmental and contextual factors affect parents, parenting behavior, and child outcomes.
4. It is important to understand the internal world of both the child and the caregiver.
5. From an infant mental health perspective, the subjective reaction of clinicians in their work with parents and infants is an important source of assessment data that can be used to foster therapeutic gains.

In the following section, we explore each of these principles and, through the use of case vignettes, the ways in which these principles can be applied to clinical work in a variety of settings.

1. *Even very young infants are understood as "social beings."* From this perspective, infant relational behavior is understood as being adaptive to particular social contexts and opportunities. Babies, if born healthy and neurologically intact, are prepared to engage in relationships. Yet

human infants remain uniquely dependent on adult caregivers for the provision of relational stimuli and opportunities. Attachment develops in the context of these caregiving relationships and reflects the kind of care provided to the infant. Interestingly, research has shown that infants are able to differentiate among caregivers, developing attachment relationships with each caregiver that are reflective of the qualities of that relationship (Cassidy & Shaver, 1999). This view of caregiver–infant relationships represents an important departure from the early view of infant bonding Klaus and Kennel (1998) in which it was understood as a unidirectional phenomenon, flowing from adult to infant. The concept of attachment relationship is bidirectional, with each partner eliciting reactions from the other. This idea is extremely important to infant mental health because it allows us to focus on important clinical questions, such as: (a) What is it like for the parent to be responsible for this particular child? (b) In what ways does this parent's caregiving style fit, or not fit, the infant's temperamental needs? (c) What situational factors (e.g., economic stress) are affecting the parent's ability to be emotionally attuned to this infant?

> Deborah and Frank are 24-year-old parents of 4-month-old Valerie. Though young and living in difficult economic circumstances, Deborah and Frank have a stable, warm relationship and are prepared to nurture and care for baby Valerie. Still, over the last 2 months, the couple shows increasing signs of strain and expresses concern that Valerie "doesn't know" them. At a well-baby check-up, the pediatrician notices that Valerie does not smile in response to visual stimuli and does not "track" visual stimuli presented to her. Further exams reveal that Valerie has serious vision deficits. While this news is difficult for Deborah and Frank, it helps them to understand their difficulty "connecting" with Valerie.

2. *Individual differences and the concept of "normal" development.* As the field of infant mental health developed, so did our understanding of the multiple pathways by which development can unfold. During the 1970s, research on infant temperament showed that infants have

a variety of temperamental styles. Rather than viewing some babies as "easy" and others as "difficult," a more important question became clear: How did the temperamental style of the infant "match" that of the parent? The concept of "goodness-of-fit" (Chess & Thomas, 1991) is important for clinicians because it focuses our attention on what a particular caregiver might find challenging about a particular infant, and conversely, how a particular caregiving style may or may not fit the temperamental needs of a specific infant. This knowledge is useful in designing interventions that focus *not* on deficits but on differences that can be addressed as strengths in the appropriate context.

Leslie W. was born full-term to adult parents. From the beginning, her parents reported feeling that Leslie "wouldn't look at" them and was happier when she was "lying on the ground next to us" but would "cry every time we picked her up." Leslie's mother had fantasized about the experience of having a baby daughter whom she would be able to hold, cuddle, bathe in a close, tactile relationship. As she came to see Leslie as not "willing" to be close to her in this way, she began to feel very rejected and even wonder if Leslie "really loved or even knew" her. Leslie and her mother were referred to an infant mental health specialist after Leslie's 4-month-old "well baby" checkup because her pediatrician was concerned that Leslie's mother was holding her at a distance and no longer making as much effort at eye contact or seeming to take much pleasure in her.

After a thorough assessment, in which Leslie's neurological status was found to be intact, the infant mental health specialist began to work with Leslie's mother on alternative ways of interacting with Leslie that did not require as much tactile stimulation but that would include eye contact and mutual gaze. Simultaneously, the infant mental health specialist gently talked with Leslie's mother, asking her to describe her feelings about the way the baby interacted and focusing on ways that Leslie behaved as her mother had imagined and also the ways in which Leslie behave differently from how her mother had imagined and hoped she would behave. By providing a forum for a nonjudgmental discussion of the loss felt by Leslie's mother in having a child who did not respond to her preferred and most comfortable way of interacting, the infant mental health specialist helped to open the door to an alternative path of relating. Several weeks later, Leslie's mother came to a session with Leslie in a stroller. Leslie's mother proudly announced that she had "something to show" the therapist and went on to gently place Leslie on the floor. Leslie's mother took out several toys and held them gently above the baby, who began to reach for the toys and displayed positive facial affect in response.

3. *Environmental factors impact parents, children, and the relationship between them.* In addition to the recognition that child development is strongly affected by the caregiving context, we also know that child development is impacted by a range of contextual factors that operate via a direct influence on development and via indirect influences through their impact on the child's family system. Economic resources, the availability of health care, education, housing, and nutrition are all important determinants of family stability and health. The availability of quality day care—a rare commodity especially among lower income families—is a critical factor in the developmental well-being of young children in the United States. It is also critical to understand the particular cultural background of a family, as social workers are well aware of, if one hopes to know the true clinical meaning and relevance of various family challenges and strengths.

Tanya is 19 years old and living on her own for the first time. Until recently, she and her 2-year-old son lived with Tanya's mother, who provided many material resources and occasional child care. Upon her graduation from high school Tanya wanted to live independently, so she found a job and an apartment. Tanya's job was full-time and with modest benefits but with very uneven work hours. Although she was able to find a subsidized child-care center relatively close to her home, it was only open from 7:30 A.M. to 6:00 P.M., Monday through Friday. However, Tanya's work hours were very unpredictable, requiring intermittent evening and weekend hours as well. When the child-care center was not operating, Tanya would leave her son with friends, neighbors, and sometimes her mother. The unpredictability of her work hours and the subsequent child-care arrangements became a stressor for her son, producing great distress on his part when he would be transferred from place to place. He became fearful and less willing to interact with others, withdrawing even from the child-care providers at the center. Although Tanya's mother offered to help in the situation, unresolved conflicts between them led Tanya to reject her offer of support. As the situation with her son's distress became more extreme, Tanya was often late to work and eventually lost her job.

From an infant mental health perspective, it would be very important to understand the meaning, to Tanya and her son, of leaving her mother's home and the subsequent relational challenges. At a time in development when safety and predictability are key, Tanya's son was feeling adrift and disconnected. How could his developmental needs be better balanced with his mother's need for independence and autonomy? Tanya's case represents an example where situational factors combine with developmental needs to create stress for both mother and child, necessitating a multipronged and possibly multigenerational solution.

4. *It is important to understand the internal world of the child and caregiver.* Prior to the work of Spitz (1944), little was understood about the psychological meaning of the caregiver to infants and young children. Since that pioneering research, clinicians and researchers have documented the active internal world of the child and the processes by which young children create, with help from their caregivers, meaning out of their experiences. Because caregiver behavior so strongly shapes the child's world, infant mental health focuses on understanding the motivation and meaning of parental behavior. Why are some parents able to take joy and pleasure in the process of caregiving, whereas others are not? What does it feel like to parent a helpless infant? What is it like to be a single parent caring for a "hard-to-soothe" infant who seems to "reject" efforts of comfort and interaction? The infant mental health perspective directs clinicians to think

about how the child is feeling, how the parent is feeling, and how the emotional state of each affects the other. This framework is not limited to the child's biological parent(s) but expands to include all caregivers with primary responsibility for the psychological and physical well-being of the child.

Infants and young children who have experienced abuse or neglect, followed by a disruption in their care and living situations, may undergo a doubly traumatic event. Peter M. was removed from his parents' care after many episodes of serious neglect. At the age of 3, Peter had often been left alone in the family's apartment for long hours at a time, with little access to food. At the time of his removal from the home, Peter was extremely withdrawn and unresponsive. His foster parents, Mr. and Mrs. T., were excited about having Peter "join their family." With no children of their own they felt that they had "a lot of love to offer" and spent a good deal of time preparing a place for Peter in their home. Upon Peter's arrival, Mr. and Mrs. T. went immediately to hug Peter and were saddened when he pulled away from them, not returning their affection. Expecting that he would settle in soon, Mr. and Mrs. T. were surprised that even though Peter certainly recognized them and showed no fear around them, he also showed no inclination to share positive affect or return any expression of affection. Indeed, every time the foster parents felt that they were making a "breakthrough" with Peter, it seemed that he would "revert back" to the more withdrawn child they had originally met.

When the caseworker came to visit the family, Mr. and Mrs. T. questioned whether Peter should remain in their home. Feeling exhausted and rejected, Mrs. T. voiced that it was "like he doesn't want me to love him." Trained in infant mental health, the caseworker was able to offer an alternative explanation to Mrs. T., stating that, for Peter, experiences of closeness and affection were associated with the painful affects of loss and anxiety. During his times alone in his family's apartment, he had coped by withdrawing into himself and "shutting down." Though the Foster parents' efforts to reach out to Peter were well intentioned and infused with affection, they had not sufficiently understood Peter's relational history and his internal working model of attachment experiences. By helping Mr. and Mrs. T. to understand Peter's behavior as a coping response, they were able to take it less personally and sustain their relationship with Peter over the length of time that was necessary for him to become more trusting in the continuity of their caring for him.

5. *How does it feel for the clinician to work with this child and family?* Clinicians who work from an infant mental health perspective have the complex task of applying their observational and conceptual skills to try and understand the emotional experience of parents and young children who often are under enormous relational and situational stress. It is important that the clinician develop skills of self-awareness in order to keep track of his or her own emotional response to the family as a whole and to the child and parent(s) as individuals. The clinician's subjective experience of the child and the family may provide important clinical data. Furthermore, because infant mental health practice is relationship based, it is important that the clinician pay attention to how each relationship he or she is forming (e.g., between the clinician and child) is impacting other relationships (e.g., between the parent and the child). The overarching goal is to improve and support the quality of the relationship between the child and his or her caregiver(s). Attaining this goal can be more difficult than it first appears because the clinician may develop strong countertransference reactions, either positive or negative, toward either the parent or the infant.

Sandra was a social worker in a community-based home-visiting program for at-risk infants and their parents. She was assigned to visit the home of Leila, a 21-year-old single mother, and her 14-month-old daughter Jasmine. Although Jasmine seemed somewhat indifferent to her mother, she was open to Sandra's overtures, handing toys back and forth to the worker and smiling when the worker spoke to her. Jasmine's mother suffered with undiagnosed and untreated depression. Her affect was generally flat and her gaze nonspecific and not directed at Jasmine. Jasmine had experienced the benefit of her grandmother's care when the grandmother would visit the apartment on a daily basis.

Sandra came to look forward to opportunities to "play with" Jasmine but began to talk less and less to Leila herself. In supervision, Sandra's mentor pointed out that, without meaning to, Sandra had begun to "leave out" the baby's mother, forming a relationship only with Jasmine and not attending to the primary goal of encouraging connection between Jasmine and Leila. At her supervisor's suggestion, Sandra began to direct Jasmine's attention to her mother (e.g., "Why don't you give that pretty toy to Mommy?") and then reward Jasmine's willingness to follow through. In addition, Sandra paid special attention to drawing Leila's attention toward even the smallest recognition paid to Leila by Jasmine (e.g., "Did you notice how she smiled when you handed her back the toy?"). In this way, Sandra took the focus off of herself and began to use herself more as a tool to help foster and kindle the connection between Jasmine and her mother.

RELATIONSHIP BASED INTERVENTION
WITH PARENTS AND INFANTS

Many different fields of practice are represented in the clinical specialty known as "infant mental health." Working in multiple contexts, infant mental health practitioners focus on strengthening the relationship between infants, young children, and their caregivers. A holistic and strengths-oriented approach, infant mental health is relevant to multiple settings, such as community-based practice, medical social work, parent–infant psychotherapy, family advocacy, and child welfare. Infant mental health clinicians are trained to recognize the multiple factors that work either to support or impede the development of health parent–child relationships. These factors include (Carter, Osofsky, & Hann, 1992; Weatherston, 2000):

- The family's need for concrete assistance and situational stability
- Parental needs for emotional support and treatment for recognized mental health issues and problems

- Parental needs for developmental guidance as to how to interpret infant behavior and anticipate the infant and young child's shifting developmental needs over time
- Early and sophisticated assessment of infant neuropsychological competency and the quality of the parent–infant relationship
- Focused and supportive parent–infant psychotherapy in cases where factors such as parental trauma and unresolved losses are impeding the parents' ability to form supportive attachment relationships with their infant
- Advocacy on behalf of vulnerable infants, children and their families

In her review of the infant mental health literature, Weatherston (2000) summarized the core skills and strategies associated with infant mental health practice. Many of these strategies were developed as the basis of relationship-focused home-visiting programs with at-risk parents and infants. It is important to remember that the clinical field of infant mental health emerged during a time of rapid progress in our understanding of the multiple competencies of the human infant *and* in our understanding of the processes by which infants and caregivers form stable relational bonds. The strategies associated with infant mental health reflect this vast body of research and, perhaps most importantly, focus attention on the emotional experience of parenthood, the psychological needs of parents, the internal world of the child, and how each of these factors influences the unfolding relationship between parent and infant in unique ways.

One of the most important contributions of infant mental health has been the commitment to a biopsychosocial view of the child in the context of the family. As a field of practice, infant mental health seeks to integrate the biopsychosocial assessment of the child "in the present" with past experiences of the caregivers, as these experiences are expressed in the parent–child relationship. Infant mental health specialists seek to connect with caregivers around current, "real-time" concerns in the parent–infant relationship and family context, while at the same time "listening for the past" as it may become represented in present-day conflicts over issues of closeness, dependency, and loss (Fraiberg, 1980; Fraiberg, Adelson, & Shapiro, 1975; Weatherston, & Buttman, 1995). This approach helps clinicians to address questions of the intergenerational transmission of family experience, itself an area of study being examined anew as researchers in the cognitive neurosciences begin to delineate the processes by which parental caretaking style and history become factors in the postnatal brain development of infants and young children (Schore, 1994).

THE INTERSECTION OF INFANT MENTAL HEALTH AND SOCIAL WORK

The core principles of infant mental health, as outlined above, derive from many fields of study and share in common a focus on facilitating infant–child development via collaborative support of the child's primary care-giving relationship(s). From a social work perspective, it is important to recognize that a child's caregiving circle may be broad, culturally diverse, and include biological parents, extended family, foster parents, child-care providers, and professionals (e.g., child welfare workers) with whom the child comes into frequent contact, and on whom the child may depend for continuity. The principles of infant mental health may be applied to each of these relationships and can be considered in the development of programs in many contexts and settings (Graham, White, Clarke, & Adams, 2001).

Social workers are likely to come into contact with families that are de-scribed as "multiproblem families." These families, although often con-cerned about the well-being of their children, may be so overwhelmed by a series of situational, individual, and family-level stressors that they are unable to foster that well-being. One of the main challenges a clinician faces is the task of forging and sustaining a working alliance, on behalf of a child, with family members who feel themselves to be "under siege" or relationally exhausted and depleted. Because a core strategy of infant mental health is to form a supportive relationship with caregivers on behalf of the child, social workers must grapple with obstacles to the working alliance. Adding to the challenge, social workers may need to work to overcome distrust that families have about "the system," especially in the field of child welfare, and because of the diverse populations with whom we work, social workers must make special and informed efforts to acknowledge and incorporate the family's cultural frame of reference into assessment and intervention planning.

Parlakian (2001) described a powerful model called "Look, Listen and Learn" that demonstrates how the use of reflective strategies can support the development of the working alliance between parent(s) and clinician and, in turn, the parent–child relationship. Each element of Parlakian's "Look, Listen and Learn" model is explored below.

The Importance of Looking

Through the use of observational skills, clinicians are able to discern important data about the child and the parent–child relationship that may be pertinent to the formulation of further intervention planning. From these nonverbal observations, clinicians can observe a lot about the neurological and physical integrity of the child and the parent, the overall mood and affect of the child and the parent, and the tenor of the parent–child relationship. The following questions form a useful observational frame:

1. Does this infant/child appear to be growing normally?
2. Is the child attaining important developmental milestones in the realms of physical, cognitive, and motor development?
3. What kind of mutual gaze or eye contact exists between caregiver and child?
4. Does the caregiver or the child appear anxious? How is this anxiety being expressed?
5. Does the caregiver appear to take pleasure in the child, displaying positive states of emotion?
6. Is the caregiver reasonably attuned and responsive to the child's signals?
7. How does it feel to you, as a clinician, to be with this caregiver and child? What does your response suggest about the overall situation?

8. Are there cultural differences or factors that are shaping your observations of this family? For example, are patterns of eye contact different from what you expect or are used to?
9. Are you, as a clinician, aware of other factors that might alter the
   way in which parent and child interact in your presence? For example, has this family had prior negative experiences with the service
   delivery system? Is the parent or caregiver depressed or utilizing
   drugs? Are there mental, emotional, or cognitive concerns about the
   parent that may alter his or her patterns of interaction?
10. Are there immediate safety concerns that need to be addressed?

The Importance of Informed "Listening"

In addition to the use of informed observations, clinicians who work
within an infant mental health perspective need to listen to the parent's
story, or narrative, with an informed understanding of those factors that are
relevant to the burgeoning attachment relationship between parent and
child. Given the depth of research on determinants of attachment quality,
clinicians must be prepared to listen for multiple sets of factors and consider how these factors may pose challenges to the caregiver–infant relationship. From a social work perspective, it is critical that we learn to listen
with a *strengths orientation*, meaning that we are in a state of *wondering*
about the meaning of the parents' statements in relation to *this individual
parent and this particular point in time*. Important questions include:

1. What themes are important to this parent/caregiver as he or she talks
   with us?
2. How is the parent feeling about the topics being discussed?
3. What seems to go easily for this parent, and what particular issues are
   stressful?
4. How does the parent understand the child's behavior? What kind of
   interpretations is the parent making?
5. Does the parent seem to see that he or she has a role in the situation?
   Does the parent have a sense of efficacy, and of being able to impact
   outcomes, on behalf of his or her children? Or does the parent seem

to feel so overwhelmed and exhausted that there is almost a sense of "learned helplessness"?

6. What is the caregiver actually saying about his or her own needs? Can you identify areas in need of concrete assistance that need to be addressed first, before more in-depth relational work can be done?

7. What basic relational skills are you able to observe and experience in conversation with this caregiver? Is there sufficient eye contact and steadiness of voice/ideas to enable a sense of connectedness and interaction? If not, do you observe this same deficit in interaction with the infant or child?

The Importance of Learning from the Baby and Caregiver

By combining the nonverbal observations gleaned from looking and the themes that emerge as relevant through the process of informed listening, clinicians are in a better position to undertake the third element of the "Look, Listen and Learn" model (Parlakian, 2001). Clinicians working from an infant mental health perspective must be able to integrate multiple sources of information and data. The nonverbal state of the infant requires the clinician to become an informed observer of infant behavior, to be able to glean important relational data from the infant's behavior and demeanor and from the quality of interaction observed between the infant and the caregiver. This keen observation, in combination with direct communication with the caregiver, can enable the clinician to formulate hypotheses about the nature of the infant–caregiver relationship, the child's overall emotional well-being, and the mental health needs of the caregiver.

INFANT MENTAL HEALTH ASSESSMENT STRATEGIES

As has been discussed, an infant mental health perspective seeks to promote healthy development for young children and their caregivers by supporting the caregiver–infant relational dyad. This perspective has applied clinical utility, as seen in the "zero-to-three" classification of relationship disorders (Zero to Three: National Center for Infants, Toddlers

& Families, 1994). Important to this classification system is the concept
that the "disorder" is specific to a particular *relationship* and is recognized via its behavioral manifestations in both the infant and caregiver.
This perspective is particularly critical in work with preverbal children,
because the clinician is able to use his or her observations of the infant
to construct a meaningful clinical formulation of the infant–caregiver
dyad.

The Look, Listen and Learn model described above incorporates
strategies designed to assess relational health in caregiver–infant dyads, in
which the clinician must attend to (1) the behavioral quality of the interaction between infant and caregiver, (2) the affective tone of the infant
and the caregiver, and (3) the degree and quality of psychological involvement of the adult caregiver with the infant, as represented in statements
that suggest how the caregiver *feels* about the child and his or her relationship with the child. These concepts are central to many models of
child mental health assessment (Greenspan & Porges, 1984). Many of
these elements are explored briefly below.

- *Behavioral quality of the interaction.* What does the clinician observe
  about the behavior of each member of the relational dyad? Given
  knowledge of developmental milestones, does the infant appear
  within the typical age range? Does the parent seem to have age-
  appropriate expectations for infant behavior? In the context of feeding or play, does the parent's behavior show concern, sensitivity, and
  organization that would serve to protect the infant from stress and
  overwhelming states of affective arousal? Does the child's behavior
  show an expectancy of comfort in interaction with the parent? Alternatively, is the child most likely to arch away from the parent or otherwise avoid interactions (e.g., a predominance of gaze aversion,
  "freezing," or withdrawal)?
- *Degree and quality of caregiver's psychological involvement.* What
  does the clinician observe about the caregiver's involvement with,
  and feelings for, the child? Every child will elicit a set of reactions
  from the caregiver based on a range of child, adult, and situational

characteristics. Is the clinician able to determine whether the caregiver's reaction is primarily positive or negative? What does the clinician understand about what it has been like, for this particular caregiver, to care for this particular child? Does the caregiver have appropriate (based on child's age) expectations of the child? What kind of attributions does the caregiver make about the child's behavior (e.g., does the caregiver overly personalize the child's behavior)? Are the attributions primarily positive (e.g., "he's curious") or negative (e.g., "He's too nosey")?

Jonathon, a full-term, healthy 11-month-old baby, was referred by his pediatrician for developmental assessment because his growth had slowed dramatically. Initial tests had ruled out organic reasons for his slowed growth, and the current working diagnosis was to rule out or confirm nonorganic failure to thrive. As part of the assessment, the infant mental health specialist was asked to observe Jonathon and his mother in both play and feeding interactions. As his mother approached him with a spoonful of food, Jonathon turned his head and made no eye contact with her. When she held him to give him a bottle, she held him away from her body, balanced precariously at the very edge of her lap. As she continued to work on feeding Jonathon, she stated that he "never seemed to want to eat," and it seemed like he was "never happy to see her" either. In the play situation, Jonathon sat on the playroom floor while his mother sat, quietly and almost motionless, next to him. Although Jonathon occasionally picked up a random toy, no eye contact was exchanged between him and his mother, and his mother made no comment about the objects in which Jonathon showed initial interest. On the few occasions that his mother did approach him, Jonathon turned his head away. As the interaction continued, Jonathon's behavior became less organized and he started to become "fussy" and to drool. Ultimately, he lay down on the play mat and closed his eyes.

What can an informed observer learn from the situation described above? First, the clinician can formulate working hypotheses that must be explored further and evaluated via the collection of additional data. However, in the above observation, several important questions immediately come to mind. First, the infant mental health specialist observes an absence of positive affect between parent and child. The "tasks" of feeding and play (central to the relational experience of infants) are conducted in an almost lifeless manner and certainly do not appear to be pleasurable to either partner. Jonathon's behavior shows no expectancy, based on past experience, that the interaction will be otherwise, and his mother states that her child "doesn't seem happy" to be around her. Behaviorally, the clinician observes a lack of physical closeness and warmth, and although Jonathon explores toys superficially, it is not with the pleasure and depth that one might expect to see in an infant his age. Over time, Jonathon's response becomes more withdrawn, until he actually lies down and closes his eyes, completely withdrawing from play and further opportunities for interaction. It is possible that Jonathon's withdrawal is a coping response that has come to characterize most of his interactions with his caregiver. In the case of nonorganic failure to thrive, this is what we often see: a baby "too tired" to sustain engagement, who withdraws from eating and play in a way that inhibits physical and social growth.

INFANT MENTAL HEALTH IN MULTIPLE CONTEXTS

Although infant mental health strategies are often used in the assessment and treatment of relational disturbances between caregivers and infants, and in infant–parent psychotherapy, the core strategies of infant mental health are relevant to many other settings and kinds of work with which social workers are familiar. As Graham and colleagues (2001) suggested, the core ideas of infant mental health can be applied to a range of programs located in different levels of the service delivery system. From a social work perspective, this flexibility is important because the quality of care received by infants and young children is relevant not only to those practitioners working with parents and infants at a microsystemic level, but also to those social workers working in areas such as prevention, child-care community organization, early intervention planning, and in broader systems such as child welfare and the courts. Graham and colleagues suggested that the core principles of infant mental be applied, in different ways, as appropriate to different settings, whenever the quality of care-giver–child relationship is a primary concern. As outlined in Graham et al., 2001, these principles may include:

1. Incorporating attachment theory into all aspects of child's assessment and treatment planning.
2. Promoting the continuity of care.
3. Providing a supportive climate for emotional development.
4. Modeling responsive caregiving.
5. Providing family support and education.
6. Identifying early signs of problems that might impede the parent–child relationship and providing additional support to families.
7. Referring for further screening or assessment as needed.

Because social workers often collaborate with professionals in allied disciplines, it is important that social work take a lead advocacy role in helping other professionals to see the ways in which the principles and strategies of an infant mental health perspective may be useful in engaging high-risk families and in developing methods of intervention that may work, across time, to support emotional development and well-being.

The primary goal of this chapter was to introduce the concept of infant mental health as an important set of principles and strategies for working with infants, young children, and the adults that comprise their circle of care. Research in the cognitive neurosciences has highlighted the importance of early intervention with young families at risk for relational disruption. Because the early years of life represent a critical period with regard to many aspects of brain development, particularly those associated with social and emotional well-being, the quality of relationships formed and sustained during this period is of critical importance. Thus, whereas the field of infant mental health began from a psychosocial perspective on the emotional needs of infants and young children, the field has now broadened to include new knowledge in the field of neurobiology that provides an important complement to our understanding of how early relational experience shapes emotional and developmental well-being.

Chapter 8

NEUROBIOLOGY APPLIED

Affect Dysregulation and Its Treatment

THE PRECEDING CHAPTER examined the ways in which strategies of prevention and early intervention can help children, whose early attachments put them at risk for later difficulties, regain a course toward adaptive and gratifying relationships throughout life. In this chapter we turn our attention to people whose life circumstances may not have afforded them the opportunities to benefit from such interventions or whose current stressors have induced affect dysregulation. Clinical social workers in many settings see clients who present with symptoms of anxiety, depression, personality disorders, posttraumatic stress reactions, or psychosis. There is increasing interdisciplinary consensus that these and other forms of psychopathology represent, in combination with constitutional vulnerabilities, problems with affect regulation secondary to troubled attachment histories (Bradley, 2000; Schore, 2003a).

Clinical curricula in schools of social work typically provide students with basic knowledge about human vulnerability and disturbance. Often this information is taught from the perspective of the *Diagnostic and Statistical Manual of Mental Disorders, Fourth Edition* (American Psychiatric

Association, 1994), or other current models for classifying types of psychopathology. These models, designed to describe disorders rather than the people with disorders, are typically atheoretical and do not attempt to account for developmental or relational factors as etiological. Supplemental materials in social work courses on this topic often include psychodynamic, cognitive-behavioral, and systems approaches to understanding the etiology of disorders. Although there is a nod in some materials toward biologically predisposing factors, scant attention is given to the role of the neurobiology of affect regulation in the development of human distress. As noted in the Introduction, we believe that the addition of this information to the social work clinician's conceptual toolbox can strengthen the underaddressed *bio* component of social work's *biopsychosocial* perspective for assessment and intervention.

As we have illustrated in earlier chapters, the study of the neurobiology of affect regulation includes a dual focus on interactions between (1) the unique features that each individual brings to lifespan development, such as genetic inheritance, constitutional predisposition, and differences in temperament; and (2) the social environment—especially the caregiving environment—in which individuals are reared. This person–environment focus fits well with current diathesis stress models of psychopathology (*diathesis* refers to constitutionally predisposing factors that render people vulnerable to difficulty; and *stress* refers to events or circumstances [stressors] that increase their vulnerability). From a neurobiological perspective, resilience, or the capacity to respond adaptively to stress, depends on attributes that potentiate the regulation of positive and negative affects. And adaptive affective regulation depends, in turn, on the integration of the various neural networks in the brain.

NEURAL NETWORK INTEGRATION

As discussed in Chapter 1, neurons form connections among themselves that result in elaborate neural networks, and these networks integrate with each other to form increasingly complex (nonlinear dynamic) neural systems. Information flows in multiple directions among these network systems. Neuroscientists divide the organization of these systems in the brain according to vertical and horizontal axes. The vertical axis includes the brainstem, limbic system, and cortex, and the horizontal axis refers to the systems comprising the left and right hemispheres.

Drawing on an impressive body of research, Cozolino (2002) proposed a model for explaining the ways in which all these systems achieve integration through efficient interconnections. *Top-down* integration links the three systems of the vertical axis, unifying the brainstem (body), limbic system (affect), and cortex (consciousness). Activation of the neural circuits moves from the top of the brain down and back up again, enabling the cortex to process, organize, or inhibit reflexes, impulses, and affects arising from the brainstem and limbic systems.

Nine-year-old Jonathan was in the fourth grade. Although he strove to be a "good student" and relate well to peers, he often failed because much of his psychological energy was directed toward containing significant free-floating anxiety. In interaction with his teacher and his parents, Jonathan often "lost it," getting very angry over mild frustrations, especially when adults were not able to come to his aid quickly enough. Ultimately, Jonathan was evaluated by a school social worker, who recognized that his anger may have been a representation of psychologically painful anxiety states. Unable to relieve his own anxiety by engaging higher-level cortical processing strategies, Jonathan looked to his parents and other trusted adults to help mitigate his anxiety. When this wish was frustrated, Jonathan's affective state overwhelmed his capacity to delay gratification, tolerate frustration, and control the unintegrated impulses arising from brainstem and limbic system stimuli.

To achieve left–right integration requires input from both left and right cerebral cortices and limbic areas for satisfactory functioning. Putting feelings into words, for example, requires integration of the cognitive and language functions of the left hemisphere and the emotional, nonverbal functions of the right. Circuits in the left hemisphere are biased toward approach behavior and positive affects, whereas those in the right are biased toward withdrawal behavior and negative affects (Bradley, 2000).

Left–right integration helps balance these biases toward adaptive neural processing and affect regulation.

> Martin, a 23-year-old graduate student in physics, came to see a clinical social worker on the recommendation of his girlfriend. She believed he was depressed and was increasingly frustrated by his seeming inability to express positive feelings toward her. From her knowledge of expressive vulnerabilities associated with insufficient left–right neural integration, the social worker hypothesized that Martin was suffering from alexithymia, a disorder that results in difficulty describing feelings and making connections between feelings, thoughts, and outward behaviors (Bradley, 2000). As part of her intervention, the social worker asked Martin to keep a daily journal in which he was to record his thoughts and feelings during the week between their appointments. This journal became the basis for discussion during sessions. In helping Martin verbally elaborate and refine the feelings appearing in the journal, the social worker hoped to foster the left–right hemispheric integration that would help him become more emotionally expressive.

When the various neural systems interconnect and intercommunicate in an integrative fashion, people are able to achieve an adaptive balance among the domains of affect, cognition, sensation, and behavior. Because neural integration fosters conscious awareness of affects and sensations, individuals are able to use what Fonagy et al. (2002) call the reflective function to become consciously aware of and regulate their feelings and sensations in ways that facilitate adaptive behavior. This capacity, in turn, presumably facilitates mentalization, the process by which people are able to attune to their own and others' mental and emotional states. If these integrative processes proceed normally during development, the outcome is *mentalized affectivity*, described as "a mature capacity for the regulation of affect and . . . the capacity to discover the subjective meanings of one's own affect states" (Fonagy et al., 2002, p. 5). This capacity also enables people to infer the mental and emotional states of others, which is central to empathic relatedness. With mentalized affectivity, people can "read" the social cues of others, reflect on the affective responses triggered in themselves, and attune their interactions accordingly.

In contrast, compromised integration puts people at risk for various disturbances in their biopsychosocial well-being and mental health, including disturbances in the reflective function that makes mentalized affectivity possible. As an example from normal development, the cognitive and emotional regression to egocentrism seen in adolescents often makes it difficult for them to take an adult perspective. They may have difficulty feeling empathy for their parents' concern for their safety when it is expressed in the imposition of a curfew. They are more likely to misinterpret this limit setting as an effort to control them.

Such misattribution of intention is also seen in "road rage:" People have been known to become dangerously enraged when they misperceive other drivers' unintentional mistakes as purposfully directed at them. At a neurobiological level they are unable to apply the reflective reasoning and impulse control associated with cortical processing to modulate the impulses emerging from limbic and brainstem regions.

In the clinical setting, we see expressions of compromised neural network integration and difficulties with mentalized affectivity in a variety of types of psychopathology. Indeed, Cozolino concluded that "psychopathology is a reflection of suboptimal integration and coordination of neural networks. Patterns of dysregulation of brain activation in specific disorders support the theory of a brain-based explanation for the symptoms of psychopathology" (2002, p. 25).

AFFECT DYSREGULATION AND PSYCHOPATHOLOGY

Inefficient, out-of-balance neural network integration can result from genetic or constitutional vulnerabilities, interactional difficulties in the early child–caregiver relationship, or extreme stress or trauma at any point in the life course. From her extensive review of research on genetic factors in the etiology of psychopathology, Bradley (2000) reported that genetic factors play a role in internalizing (anxiety and mood) disorders, externalizing (disruptive behavior) disorders, and psychosis, all displaying signs and symptoms of affect dysregulation. The considerable influence

of genetic factors notwithstanding, the degree of their influence is mediated by environmental factors.

Schore, for example, pointed out that opioids, corticosteroids, and other
gene-regulating hormones are influenced by interactions with the external environment, especially the social environment, during the sensitive
period of early caregiving during which connections in the infant's limbic
system are proliferating at a high rate; changes in the social environment,
in turn, activate genetic programs in the "microarchitecture of growing
brain regions" (2003a, p. 33), thus playing a role in shaping each person's
neuropsychological internal environment. As Cozolino put it, the brain's
"neural architecture comes to reflect the environment that shapes it"
(2002, p. 22). When the social environment is either chronically stressful
and overstimulating or lacking in sufficient stimulation and challenge,
hormonal and neurotransmitter changes in the brain can induce cell
death in the affective areas of the limbic system, leading to affect dysregulation and compromised neural network integration. There is general consensus among neuroscientists that the region of the limbic system most
involved in these processes is the right orbitofrontal cortex (Bradley, 2000;
Cozolino, 2002; Schore, 1994, 2003a, 2003b).

Numerous clinician-scholars have employed findings from research
on the neurobiology of affect regulation to help explain the etiology of
borderline personality disorder (see Cozolino, 2002; Fonagy et al., 2002;
Schore, 2003a). The impulsivity, instability in interpersonal relations,
identity confusion, intense anger, feelings of emptiness, difficulty being
alone, and self-destructive behaviors seen in clients with this disorder are
believed to reflect a combination of constitutional vulnerabilities and
traumatic early experiences with caregivers that led to a disorganized attachment style. This combination of risk factors appears to compromise
neural network integration in ways that challenge the capacity for reflective thinking and mentalized affectivity. Clients with borderline personality disorder tend to misinterpret the relational cues of those with whom
they attempt intimate relationships. They misidentify, disregard, or bypass these cues and instead distort their perception of the mental states of
others through such defensive maneuvers as splitting and projective identification. A simple criticism can be experienced as total rejection and

abandonment, triggering rageful revenge or self-destructive acts. Clients with these vulnerabilities present formidable clinical challenges in that they often communicate how how they feel, not in language, but by projectively inducing their angry, empty, or disorganized feelings in their clinicians.

It is important to emphasize that not all mental health issues addressed by clinical social workers are associated with early difficulties in neural network integration and affect dysregulation. Clearly the brain is highly susceptible to these vulnerabilities during the sensitive periods of infancy and early childhood. But chronic stress or acute trauma at any point in the life cycle can disrupt information processing in ways that challenge the neural network integration and adaptive affect regulation of previously well-functioning individuals. Adults subjected to trauma, for example, may develop dissociative symptoms reflective of disconnections among the neural networks involved with cognition, emotion, sensation, and behavior. Such symptoms can consolidate into states of chronic arousal, intrusion, and avoidance, typically seen in posttraumatic stress disorder (Maxmen & Ward, 1995).

As noted in the Introduction, recent scholarship has begun to elaborate the neurobiological basis for the way in which psychotherapy can enhance neural network integration and its associated adaptive affect regulation. The most concise and approachable explanatory framework is Cozolino's 2002 book, *The Neuroscience of Psychotherapy: Building and Rebuilding the Human Brain*. In what follows, we employ his framework as a structure for describing how clinical intervention works.

BASIC PRINCIPLES OF CLINICAL INTERVENTION

Cozolino asserted that "all forms of therapy, regardless of theoretical orientation, will be successful to the degree to which they foster neural growth and integration" (2002, p. 27). As described earlier, the neural networks involved include those dedicated to sensation (associated with the brainstem), affect (associated with the limbic system), cognition (associated with the cortex), and behavior. Neuronal growth and network integration are enhanced in clinical work through (1) the provision of a "holding environment" involving a safe and trusting relationship; (2) the acquisition of new information and experience across neural network domains; (3) either simultaneous or alternating activation of neural networks that are dissociated or insufficiently integrated; (4) the induction of moderate levels of stress—what Cozolino calls *safe emergencies*—alternating with episodes of safety and calm reflection; (5) the use of clinically co-constructed narratives that integrate cognition with affective and bodily experience; and (6) the processing of the new experiences emerging from therapy in ways designed to continue further posttherapy growth and integration.

Cozolino (2002) suggested that, regardless of theoretical orientation, clinicians facilitate achievement of these objectives through techniques ranging from (1) psychoeducation to (2) encouraging clients to risk and practice new behaviors and ways of thinking, to (3) interpretations designed to make clients aware of unconscious feelings and impulses, to (4) cognitive strategies designed to enhance the integration between thoughts and feelings. If successful, these strategies help clients acquire levels of affect tolerance and regulation that enable them to maintain their gains and continue their growth after termination. One promising intervention approach to borderline personality disorder based on these strategies is dialectical behavior therapy (DBT), originated by Marsha Linehan (1993). This integrative intervention, which includes behavioral contracting to ensure safety, psychoeducation, cognitive restructuring, individual relationship-based therapy, and group experiences, is designed to foster a capacity to reflect more realistically on others' behavior, manage strong affects and impulses more effectively, and try out new, more reality-based relationships.

One of the implicit ways clients internalize an enhanced capacity for affect tolerance and regulation is by observing how the clinician responds to their distress. For example, by responding in a calm, soothing, tolerant, and modulated manner to the dysregulated affect of a client in crisis, the attuned clinician models a different way of managing strong emotion. Using Fonagy and associates' (2002) concept of *markedness* as applied to caregiver–infant affect mirroring, the clinician empathically reflects back the essential characteristics of the client's affect (e.g., a frown, a nonverbal utterance of concern), but at a more moderate, regulated pitch than that displayed by the client.

It is important to note that these regulatory transactions occur primarily in nonverbal, prosodic, and gestural ways. Neither clinician nor client is consciously aware of them. Most of the empathic resonance occurs during gaze transactions exchanged in split-second intervals. Repeated episodes of such transactions enable the client gradually to calm down enough to begin to put the strong affects into words. Once this process begins, the clinician can help the client expand on his or her descriptions of the problem, toward the development of *integrative narratives* (Cozolino, 2002). These narratives foster an integration of cognition and affect in ways that enable both partners in the dialogue to consciously process the client's distress and develop plans for addressing it. In other words, cortical processes are enlisted to moderate the affective arousal generated by subcortical (limbic, brainstem) neural networks, while affective (right-brain) arousal is balanced by cognitive (left-brain) processing. Cozolino concluded that "narratives co-constructed with therapists provide a new template for thoughts, behaviors, and ongoing integration" (2002, p. 26).

The language of these narratives apparently exerts a powerful integrative effect on neural networks throughout the brain. At about 18 months, the language centers of the left hemisphere enter their sensitive period of rapid development (Pally, 2000). These "interpreter" centers begin to exert their motivational drive to understand and explain in a linear, cause-and-effect manner the nonlinear, context-dependent, imagistic information generated in the right hemisphere. This interhemispheric integration facilitates the development of coherent narratives (Siegel, 1999). As this integration evolves, autobiographical memory makes it possible for children to begin to forge cognitive connections between places, events, and the self across time. They are told stories and begin to tell them, describing interactions that integrate sensations, affects, thoughts, and behaviors toward a coherent life story and consolidated self-identity.

Narratives are, by definition, interpersonal processes. As caregivers engage their children in dialogues that focus on their thoughts, feelings, perceptions, and desires, they both strengthen the security of attachment and facilitate children's neural network integration. In this process, a level of communication best described as interpersonal resonance occurs. Logical, linear, verbal communication promotes left hemisphere–left hemisphere resonance, while tone of voice, gestures, facial expressions, and other aspects of nonverbal communication enhance right hemisphere–right hemisphere resonance. As they co-construct stories related to their inner lives and their lives together, the securely attached caregiver and child achieve bilateral-to-bilateral resonance that advances neural network integration in both partners (Siegel, 1999).

By extension, the success of the clinical process also depends on the achievement of interpersonal resonance between client and clinician. With clients who bring histories of insecure attachments, trauma, or chronically stressful life situations, the goals of intervention include displaying emotional attunement, fostering affect regulation, and coconstructing narratives toward the goal of neural network integration. Although neuroscientists suggest that all forms of clinical intervention share these goals, different therapies emphasize different means of achieving them. We turn now to brief reviews of the neurobiological substrates of psychodynamic, cognitive-behavioral, and systems interventions.

PSYCHODYNAMIC INTERVENTIONS

In its first iteration, Freud's "talking cure" focused on rendering unconscious impulses, affects, and cognitions conscious so as to enable clients to have more choice about, and mastery over, their expression. With the development of his structural theory (Freud, 1923/1961), this goal was augmented by that of enhancing ego functions and strengthening adaptive defenses toward the goal of reducing anxiety secondary to conflict between primitive drives (id) and the moral imperatives associated with civilization (superego). With the advent of object relations theory, attachment theory, and self psychology, attention turned to the mutative power of the therapeutic relationship. The assumption of these latter approaches is that new relational experiences with an attuned clinician can repair misattunements and difficulties with affect regulation derived from compromised attachments in early childhood. Given social work's emphasis on the helping relationship as central to effective intervention, the "relational" perspectives of object relations/attachment theory and self psychology provide the best fit with the profession's philosophy and objectives (Applegate, 2004).

Regardless of emphasis, psychodynamic theories cohere around several basic assumptions: (1) the existence of both a conscious and an unconscious mind; (2) the importance of early childhood development in determining mental health or psychopathology; and (3) the role of defenses in helping people regulate affects and enhance coping strategies. In translating these assumptions into the language of neuroscience, Cozolino (2002) suggested that psychodynamic theory addresses the disjunctions and dissociations between the neural networks of conscious and unconscious processing and between conscious awareness and unconscious derivatives of past experience. He viewed defenses as the manner in which neural networks become organized to diminish the anxiety and depression associated with attachment difficulties in early development. Mature defenses such as intellectualization, sublimation, and humor help people maintain reality testing, adaptive relationships, and creative outlets for unacceptable impulses, with minimal distortion of reality. Less mature defenses such as denial, projection, and dissociation distort reality to the degree that they impair people's functional and relational capacities. Because most defenses are organized in subcortical "hidden layers" of neural processing, they remain largely unconscious.

Psychodynamic clinicians try to establish conditions in which clients can transfer onto them the unconscious implicit memories and expectations of relationships with significant others, referred to as mental representations (Bradley, 2000). These mental representations are, at the neurobiological level, the schemas or internal working models organized in the neural networks of the social brain. The transference process activates these neural networks of representations and expectations and brings them to life in the clinical relationship so that they can be modified toward resolution of conflict and improved affect regulation (Westen & Gabbard, 2002). Because the clinical process challenges the client to relinquish familiar ways of coping with uncomfortable affects, the client invariably resists awareness of the meaning of unconscious defenses and dysfunctional ways of thinking and behaving.

As resistance is examined and worked through via clarification, confrontation, and interpretation, clients gain greater conscious awareness of how their minds work. They can try on more adaptive ways of thinking and behaving with the support of a new attachment figure, thus altering mental representations of themselves in relation to others. At the neurological level, this process facilitates top–down and right–left neural network integration (Cozolino, 2002). This integration, in turn, enhances the reflective function necessary for mentalization and affect regulation (Fonagy et al., 2002).

COGNITIVE–BEHAVIORAL INTERVENTIONS

Cognitive–behavioral interventions focus on the role of people's thoughts, appraisals, and beliefs in determining their feelings and behaviors. Clinicians emphasizing this approach contend that inaccurate appraisals of situations lead to dysfunctional thinking, which, in turn, generates affect dysregulation. In recursive fashion, the dysregulation of affect further interrupts processes of rational cognitive appraisal. The difficulties primarily addressed by cognitive–behavioral approaches are those related to anxiety and depression.

In clients with obsessive–compulsive symptoms, phobias, panic disorder, or other anxiety disorders, the affect of fear impairs the accurate appraisal of situations in ways that inhibit and distort reality testing. In those with depression, negative affect fosters a pessimistic view of themselves, the world, and the future. From a neuroscience perspective, the therapeutic goal is to promote conscious control of cognitions and affects by enhancing the linear, language-based cortical processes of the left hemisphere while inhibiting or regulating the nonlinear, preverbal, and imagistic processes of the negatively biased right hemisphere and subcortical regions (Cozolino, 2002). In working with depression, for example, clients are encouraged to engage in positive "self-talk" designed to counteract automatic negative thinking. For clients with anxiety, clinicians provide education about its physiological symptoms (e.g., hyperventilation, elevated heart rate), set up situations designed to gradually expose and desensitize them to feared stimuli, and teach relaxation training to help them control their level of arousal during exposure. Research findings document that such strategies bring about alterations in brain functioning (Schwartz et al., 1996, as cited in Cozolino, 2002).

Traditionally, cognitive–behavioral approaches have deemphasized the role of the therapeutic relationship in fostering change. But recently there has been greater emphasis in these approaches on the relational processes that facilitate them. Clinicians practicing on the basis of these newer conceptualizations recognize that an accepting, attuned, nonjudgmental therapeutic relationship plays a part in reworking maladaptive cognitive schemas (Bradley, 2000).

SYSTEMS INTERVENTIONS

Systemic or interactional interventions such as couple and family therapy seek to alter maladaptive interactions so as to make them less aversive and more mutually reinforcing. When successful, these interventions reduce interpersonal tensions and negative affects by altering systemic patterns of affect regulation. These approaches proceed from the knowledge that neural networks are first sculpted by early interactions with the social environment. As reviewed earlier, infant–caregiver pre-attachment and attachment interactions are organized and encoded neurally into networks of sensory, motor, and affective learning. Resulting mental representations, or schemas, of the self in interaction with others extert a powerful influence on subsequent attachments people form later in life. Because in this sense the brain is socially organized, clinicians employing systems interventions believe that working with the social system in which the client is engaged offers unique opportunities to modify dysfunctional attachment schemas.

Patterns of dysregulated affect in family systems may lead to the scapegoating of one family member, often a child, in ways that compromise his or her mental health. As systems theorists conceptualize it, this process unconsciously induces the family scapegoat either to "contain" (internalize) or act out (externalize) anxiety, depression, or other distressing affects so as to reduce them in other family members. Although ostensibly more comfortable with this unconscious arrangement, the others in the family are dependent on the scapegoat to regulate their affect; they thereby compromise their own internal capacities for affect regulation. This dysfunctional pattern, over time, becomes encoded in the neural architecture of all family members, who sustain it in order to experience a sense of safety. Children emerging from these family systems, in turn, are likely to choose partners who enable them to recreate the dysfunctional family-of-origin dynamics. As Cozolino put it, "The problems of each family are determined through a series of successive childhoods; it is a multigenerational unconscious shaping of neural structure passed on from generation to generation" (2002, p. 58).

For such families, systems interventions attempt to engage each member in the process of becoming aware of the warded off, projected affects and the manner in which they have shaped family dynamics. This process begins with psychoeducation about how systems operate and exploration of the history of both sides of the family across generations. The goal is to reduce high levels of distressing affect to moderate levels in order to facilitate each participant's neural network integration. Learning and practicing new patterns of communication, assertiveness training, and cooperation "increase cortical involvement with previously reflexive and regressive emotion and behaviors" (Cozolino, 2002, p. 59). With these skills, each member of the family system learns to take responsibility for his or her own affects in ways that foster neural and psychosocial integration.

COMMON FACTORS AMONG INTERVENTIONS

Neuroscientifically informed clinicians agree that all forms of intervention share the common goal of promoting affect regulation (Bradley, 2000; Cozolino, 2002; Schore, 1994, 2003b). All of them emphasize the importance of experiences intended to expose clients to previously avoided situations in the context of the "holding environment" of an accepting, nonjudgmental helping relationship. In psychodynamic interventions, painful affects are evoked in the transference as clients recall and reexperience hurts and disappointments from early childhood. In cognitive–behavioral interventions, clients are invited to confront the anxiety or depression with which they have coped by avoiding feared situations or clinging to irrational beliefs. In systems interventions, clients are asked to become aware of the distressing unconscious affects that have led to patterns of projection and dysfunctional communication in their intimate relationships.

The support and encouragement of an empathically attuned clinician helps keep the uncomfortable affects aroused in the intervention process at moderate rather than overwhelming levels. This moderating function is crucial, in that high levels of arousal inhibit cortical processing, whereas moderate levels facilitate it. Fostering the capacity to tolerate and regulate affects that have previously been warded off through unconscious defenses or conscious coping strategies of inhibition and avoidance is central to all forms of clinical intervention. More modulated affects make it possible for clients to engage less reflexively and more reflectively in the clinical encounter. Once less affectively dysregulated, they are able to participate in the coconstruction of narratives, with the clinician, that strengthen their capacity for explicit, autobiographical memory and offer new, more reality-based perspectives on themselves and their lives. These narratives, at the neurobiological level, facilitate top–down and left–right neural network integration—a biological prerequisite for continued postintervention growth and well-being (Cozolino, 2002).

CLINICAL INTERVENTION AND NEURAL PLASTICITY

The hypothesis that psychotherapeutic interventions contribute to neural network integration is based on the assumption that neurons possess the ability to change the way they behave and interconnect in response to environmental stimuli. Research conducted with both animal and human subjects has demonstrated the neural plasticity of the brain, or its ability to forge new synaptic connections, and thus rewire itself, even into adult midlife (Black, Jones, Nelson, & Greenough, 1997; Cozolino, 2003; Schwartz & Begley, 2002). Neural plasticity is experience-dependent; as

Begley put it, "The brain is dynamic, and the life we lead leaves its mark in the complex circuitry of the brain—footprints of the experiences we have had, the thoughts we have thought, and actions we have taken" (2002, p. B4). Regions that get the most use are those most likely to endure and expand; recall that those neurons that fire together wire together (Hebb, 1949). By extension, neurobiologically oriented clinicians suggest that the focal influences of clinical intervention can draw on neural plasticity to modify the brain's synaptic architecture.

THE INTEGRATIVE NATURE OF CLINICAL SOCIAL WORK PRACTICE

Because they work in such a variety of practice settings—from child welfare agencies, to hospitals, to mental health clinics, to private practice—clinical social workers are trained and called upon to marshal skills from all three of the methods of intervention described above. Although some specialize more in one than another of the methods, clinical social workers tend to integrate aspects of all of them in the diverse, often unpredictable and multisystemic professional episodes in which they become engaged. The conceptual basis of this integration, as described in the Introduction, is social work's emphasis on the mutative power of the helping relationship. Indeed, decades of accumulated practice wisdom have strengthened social workers' conviction that the client's *affective experience* of the clinical relationship is the factor determining the effectiveness of any form of intervention.

The interpersonal matrix of this affective experience is composed of both implicit (emotional, procedural) and explicit (cognitive, verbal, declarative) dimensions of interaction. The implicit dimension acts as the "music" behind the words of explicit interactions. Expressed in contingent facial mirroring, gestures, eye contact and moments of gaze aversion, shared postures, and prosodic utterances, the implicit dimension operates at a nonconscious level but exerts a constant, moment-to-moment organizing and regulatory influence on both parties. The conscious, verbal behaviors of listening and speaking are typically more intermittent. While engaging in these behaviors, client and clinician are continually influencing each other's duration of utterance, intonation, timing, body language, and level of affective arousal. The emotional and procedural dimensions of clinical communication are analogous to infant–caregiver communication.

Beebe and Lachmann (2002) proposed three organizing principles to describe the dynamics of this communication and the manner in which it finds expression in both infant–caregiver and client–clinician interactions. (1) According to the *principle of ongoing regulation*, the interacting partners experience a sense that they are affectively "in tune" with each other. Through the rhythms of their interactions, they learn to expect certain kinds of responses to their affective displays. These expectancies become part of their regulatory repertoire. (2) According to the *principle of disruption and repair*, the partners inevitably fall "out of tune" at different junctures. Because contingent interactions feel positive and misattuned interactions feel negative, the pair will make attempts to "repair" the misattunement. As noted, these sequences of attunement, misattunement, and reattunement are inevitable; and the experience of successfully reattuning out-of-tune interactions generates a sense of confidence that disruptions can be safely repaired. (3) Finally, according to the *principle of heightened affective moments*, patterns of interaction are further organized during interactive episodes during which one or both partners experience a transformation, positive or negative, of their state of arousal, affect, and cognition.

Neurobiological theory suggests that, as with infants and caregivers, these processes of mutual regulation affect neural network organization in the client–clinician pair. Recall, for example, that various facial expressions are associated with particular physiological states. The perception of positive or negative emotion in each partner generates a resonant affective state in the other. As each partner's face and mirror neurons become activated, there is believed to be a simultaneous reorganization of networks in the right orbitofrontal cortex, the brain's affective core (Cozolino, 2002; Schore, 1994).

This biopsychosocial integration offers a rigorously conceptualized and research-based explanatory framework for understanding how the clinical relationship works. For social work, this formulation validates and privileges the quiet, sustaining, and supportive relational backdrop to the range of interventions, from assisting individual clients with emotional problems, to advocating with others on their behalf, to gaining the cooperation of others toward modifying aspects of clients' external environments. The emphasis on attachment dynamics as key to successful intervention puts as much, if not more, emphasis on the experience of "being with" the client than on "doing for" him or her. This element of successful helping efforts has always been part of social work's practice wisdom; adding the neurobiological dimension further strengthens and affirms this wisdom.

A CAUTIONARY NOTE

Because the conceptualization of the clinical relationship proposed here is an elaboration of communication patterns studied in infant–caregiver pairs, there is a troubling tendency to undertake clinical work based on these ideas in a manner that is best characterized as "reparenting." This literal approach can seem particularly compelling in episodes of support- ive work with traumatized or crisis-ridden clients, whose regression and confusion may make them appear childlike. Although it can be argued that derivatives of earliest infant–caregiver attachment dynamics exist in client–clinician interactions, to set out to replicate them represents a mis- understanding and misapplication of theory.

Such an approach proceeds from potentially dangerous assumptions: One is that the early caregivers in the client's life did a poor job; another is that the clinician can do a better job (Applegate, 1993). These assump- tions fail to account for factors such as the client's own constitutional vulnerabilities and temperament, the complexity of clients' postinfancy cognitive and symbolic capacities, stress-inducing social–environmental conditions during early life, and stresses and traumas originating in adult development. Furthermore, these assumptions can promote fantasies of clinical omnipotence that can result in the misuse of the clinician's au- thority in ways that disempower the client. Finally, the assumptions re- flect a deficit model of assessment and intervention that is in conflict with social work's commitment to a strengths-based approach that honors client agency, competence, and resilience.

With these caveats in mind, we turn now to an examination of specific types of mental health vulnerabilities presented by families typically seen in clinical social work settings. Using detailed case studies, we illustrate how clinical social workers might apply knowledge of the neurobiology of affect regulation and neural network integration to various approaches to assessment and intervention.

Chapter 9

THREE CASE STUDIES

THE FIRST CASE ILLUSTRATES a psychodynamic approach that incorporates concepts from object relations theory, attachment theory, and the psychoneurobiology and intergenerational transmission of early trauma. Also illustrated are the impact of relational trauma on memory, the reflective function, and neural network integration. The case demonstrates ways in which the repair of relational disruptions in treatment can enhance adaptive affect expression and regulation.

TAMARA: A CASE FROM CHILD WELFARE

Nineteen-year-old Tamara, an African-American single mother, was referred to Children and Youth Services (CYS) of the Department of Public Welfare by a city hospital emergency room nurse practitioner who was making arrangements for Tamara's 2-year-old daughter, Hope, to be treated for a broken arm. While examining Hope, the nurse practitioner had noticed bruises on her legs, shoulders, and back. Asking Tamara to wait in the waiting room, the nurse practitioner consulted with the on-call pediatrician, and together they decided to make a report of suspected abuse. They also followed the hospital policy requiring them to admit Hope as a protective measure, until suspicions of possible child abuse could be investigated and arrangements could be made for her safety, if needed. When the CYS social worker assigned to the case telephoned the nurse practitioner to obtain more information, she learned that Tamara would be returning to the hospital the next afternoon to talk further with the nurse and the pediatrician, so she made arrangements to meet Tamara there.

During this phone call, the nurse practitioner warned the social worker that Tamara was "hell on wheels." While Hope was being examined, Tamara had been antagonistic, loudly argumentative, and uncooperative, appearing to regard Hope's injury as "no big deal." The next day, as the social worker prepared to meet Tamara, she began to feel anxious, knowing that her task of beginning to form a working relationship with Tamara would be a formidable challenge, given that she was a Caucasian woman representing an agency often viewed by people in Tamara's housing project as unfeelingly wresting children from their families. The social worker became aware of mental images of an angry young woman belligerently demanding that she take Hope home immediately. The social worker mused that Tamara might have similar mental pictures of the worker—as punitive, demanding, and dismissive—fearing a stranger who might take her daughter away from her. These insights helped the worker feel more empathy for Tamara and better prepared her to begin the process of engagement.

Entering the interview cubicle where Tamara waited, the social worker encountered a grim-looking but quite beautiful young woman gazing up at the television monitor. When the social worker introduced herself, Tamara remained silent and kept her eyes on the TV. The social worker asked if she might sit down. Tamara, picking up a can of diet soda but keeping her eyes glued on the TV, finally said, "Whatever. Suit yourself." Taking a seat, the worker looked for a way to engage Tamara. Trying not to sound too effusive, she commented, "I like your sweater. It looks just right for a cold day like this." Tamara snapped back, "Look, I'm not here for small talk—I just want to get Hope and go home. We have a long bus ride. Why don't you do whatever you're supposed to do. Me? I'm going to the main lobby until you're done." With that she stood up and headed toward the door. Instantly, the social worker knew that, by making a comment about Tamara's appearance, she had moved too close to a young woman who needed to protect herself by keeping an adversarial distance.

Remaining seated, the worker said, "You know, you did the right thing by bringing Hope in yesterday. You were right to think that her injury needed immediate attention. I know how much you'd like to take her home, but I think the nurse explained that the hospital is required to keep her until we have a clearer picture of what happened. You're welcome to come see her tomorrow. You've had an exhausting afternoon here, but we do need to talk a little more about Hope—then you can go home. I'll arrange for your bus fare." Making momentary eye contact for the first time, Tamara glared at the worker. "Well, I don't have all night." The worker registered the anger in Tamara's face, but considered her brief glance a promising development. Noticing that the she looked wary about reentering the cubicle, the worker suggested they go to the cafeteria, a more relaxed and less confining area.

Tamara was restless and fidgety as they sat in the cafeteria. She continued to avert her eyes from the social worker's face, looking out the window or down at her lap. Attempting to forge some connection, the worker asked Tamara where she lived and about her bus trip to the hospital the preceding day. When the worker learned that Tamara lived in a distant housing project and had transferred to three different buses to get there, the worker said, "That must have been terrible, with Hope in pain and difficult to manage. I wonder if it would have been easier to call 911?" Bristling, Tamara shot back, "Yeah, right. You never know when they're going to show up, and they're too nosey when they do!" The worker translated this assertion as a message to her that people who are supposed to help are too intrusive and cannot be trusted.

Recognizing that Tamara needed to preserve her distancing tactics and could not be expected to warm up at this early point in their relationship, the social worker moved to the less intimate process of gathering basic factual information. Tamara maintained her distance, but did provide the needed information. The worker learned that Hope was Tamara's only child, that she had recently lost her job at a fast food restaurant, and was receiving public assistance. When the worker asked about others in her extended family, Tamara appeared surprised and called a halt—"I don't know why you need to know that stuff. This is just about Hope and me." Retreating, the worker decided to postpone this inquiry. She continued, "You're right—that is our main concern. I wonder if you could tell me what happened?" Tamara replied, "Well! Finally somebody asked *me*! It's real simple—she was playing on the landing out front of our building, and one of the older kids pushed her down the stairs." The worker did not question this version of Hope's injury but said that, because the emergency room staff had reported it, they would need to investigate the situation further. Hope would remain in the hospital a couple of days but would then be placed in temporary foster care until the investigation was complete.

With this, Tamara launched into a tirade against the hospital, CYS, and, most vociferously, the social worker's incompetence. The social worker, feeling attacked, frightened, and defensive, took a few moments to calm herself and imagined that her own feelings might be mirroring Tamara's. She said, "It sounds like you're feeling that we can't be helpful and that you're being blamed unfairly for not being a good mother. But I know that, because you brought Hope in for treatment, you have her best interests at heart. Even though you may not be able to trust that anything good can come of this, I want you to know that I'll do everything I can to make sure we don't let you down, as others may have. From what you've told me, you've been having a rough time of it even before Hope's injury. Perhaps over the next few weeks, while Hope is in foster care, we can talk about what you've been going through." Tamara did calm down a bit, but angrily declared that she would be coming to the hospital to see Hope and couldn't be expected to go to that "that welfare office." The worker told her that she would also be at the hospital the next day, and Tamara grudgingly agreed to another meeting in the cafeteria.

The social worker was assigned to a unit of CYS wherein she was able to provide intensive services to families such as Tamara's. This service made it possible for her to carry few cases and to see them as often as as needed. Recognizing that many families referred to the agency presented problems stemming from attachment vulnerabilities, staff members made establishing a trustworthy therapeutic holding environment the first priority of their interventions. With this in mind, the social worker began to form a relationship with Tamara. She recognized that she would have to be alert and respond sensitively to Tamara's need to set the pace, if initial engagement were to proceed to a working alliance.

Tamara failed to appear for their next cafeteria meeting. When the social worker telephoned her that afternoon, Tamara said she had "better things to do" after visiting Hope. The worker said that she would like to stop in during visiting hours to see Hope and perhaps she and Tamara could go to the cafeteria afterward. Hope replied icily, "Well, all right. If you've not got anything better to do with your time." The worker mused that this remark probably reflected Tamara's sense that she was not important enough to merit the worker's attention.

When the social worker dropped into Hope's room the next day, she found Tamara playing and talking with her and noted that Hope was responding to her mother with animation. When it was time to leave, the worker was struck by the warmth of Tamara's goodbye and the longing look in Hope's eyes. In the elevator on the way downstairs, Tamara fell quiet once again and appeared withdrawn. The worker remarked, "You have a beautiful little girl. It must be very hard leaving her here." Tamara's features softened a bit, but she said nothing.

The social worker learned later in the week that a complete pediatric and neurological evaluation of Hope revealed that, with the exception of some speech delay, her development was proceeding normally. She had warmed up quickly to her primary nurse and the pediatrician, suggesting to the worker that her attachment history had not been chronically traumatic. Tamara visited Hope each day, and staff on her floor remarked about the loving quality of their interactions. The results of Hope's evaluation and these observations led the social worker to feel that reunification of mother and daughter was a strong possibility. Meanwhile, the worker made arrangements for foster care and set up a meeting in which Tamara could meet the foster mother—a warm, personable woman who was one of the agency's most experienced foster parents. This meeting marked a small turning point in the case—Tamara seemed surprised that the worker had included her in it. The worker also took care to arrange for Tamara to have frequent visits with Hope. From this point on, Tamara's typically angry facial expression softened a bit and she seemed slightly more open and approachable.

When Hope was discharged from the hospital, the social worker suggested to Tamara that their next meetings could be at Tamara's home. Again, Tamara registered surprise: "You mean, I won't be seeing someone else?" Instantly the social worker realized that part of Tamara's guarded reluctance to begin a relationship with her was that she was expecting to be transferred to another worker. The worker hypothesized that this expectation of a short-lived relationship possibly derived from tenuous and transitory attachment bonds earlier in her life. Assuring Tamara that she would continue to work with her, the social worker arranged the first of many home visits.

For that first visit, the social worker arrived at Tamara's apartment door at the appointed time. It soon became apparent that Tamara was not at home—or was not answering her door. When the social worker got back to her office, she telephoned Tamara to set up another time. When she reminded Tamara of their appointment, Tamara nonchalantly said, "Oh, yeah. I guess I just forgot. I had to run down to the grocery and just got back." The social worker, tired after a long and stressful day, experienced an almost visceral flare of anger and, without thinking, curtly replied, "Well, I hope you can do better next time—I had to cancel some other things in order to get there today." With that, Tamara abruptly slammed down the phone.

Instantly, the social worker felt remorseful over losing her temper with Tamara. She spent several minutes reflecting on her behavior and began to wonder if she had become involved in an enactment with Tamara that replicated Tamara's earlier experiences with helpers. It was likely that Tamara was testing the worker's resolve to stay in the relationship, and the worker had failed the test. In addition, by setting up circumstances so that the worker would find her absent, Tamara may have been giving the worker an experience of what it had been like for her to be left alone. Knowing that she needed to repair this disruption in their relationship, the social worker called back and apologized for her behavior. She said, "I guess I felt disappointed and let down that we couldn't meet, and my feelings got the best of me. I imagine that's a way you've felt at times, too. Maybe you weren't sure I'd even show up. I wonder if we can schedule another time tomorrow." Tamara was silent a few moments then softly replied, "Whatever."

The following day Tamara was at home at the appointed time. She did not reply to the social worker's greeting as she opened the door, but did motion for her to come in and take a seat. The social worker noted to herself the tidiness of the apartment, including an immaculate and cheerfully decorated child's room, presumably Hope's. Tamara took a chair on the other side of the room and turned her attention to a program on the television. When the social worker wondered if she might turn the TV off so they could talk, Tamara muted the sound but left the picture on. As the social worker tried to engage Tamara in conversation, Tamara either shrugged or gave monosyllabic answers, glancing periodically at the TV and only momentarily making eye contact. Assuming that Tamara's offputting behavior was a way of managing her affect, the worker took care to modulate her own affective tone so as not to increase her client's discomfort further. Yet the worker could not shake her sense of disconnection and discouragement when she left.

This strained interactional pattern characterized their meetings over the next several home visits, usually scheduled twice a week. By the fourth one, the worker began to wonder if she would ever forge a trusting relationship with Tamara. At one point she found herself feeling the urge to give up on her. Identifying this impulse as a likely sign of countertransference to Tamara's transferential expectation that those in helping roles would give up on her, the worker said, "I'm not sure about this—but I'm wondering if you're expecting that I'm going to be like others who have let you down. You seem to be keeping your guard up in anticipation of that happening, as it may have with others in your life. It may seem hard to tell me what's been going on right now, but I'm willing to wait until you're ready." Silent for several moments, Tamara finally sighed and mumbled, "Talking doesn't do any good—sometimes it just makes things worse." Asked to elaborate, Tamara did not reply. She was silent for the remainder of the visit, but the social worker was encouraged that she had shared as much as she did and felt a slight tempering in the emotional climate between them.

Meanwhile, the visits between Tamara and Hope were going well; it was obvious to the social worker and the foster mother that they had a strong positive connection. By the sixth home visit, the social worker noticed that, when she smiled at Tamara, she could detect a tentative half-smile in return. Tamara was beginning to answer questions more responsively, though she seemed to have difficulty putting feelings into words. Gradually, however, her story unfolded—at first in a fragmented, disjointed, and affectless manner. To help lend coherence to Tamara's narrative, the social worker would interject, "I wonder if we could back up a bit—I'm not sure I understand the order of when these things happened" or "And who else was there when that happened?" In doing so, she was consciously helping Tamara organize the bits and pieces of her history. In tandem with Tamara's slowly increasing openness, the social worker felt more affectively alive, nodded more frequently, uttered nonverbal responses to the story, and frequently noticed that she was sitting in a manner similar to Tamara's. Although not always a smooth process, the pair appeared to be finding an interactional rhythm, both unaware of doing so.

With sensitive inquiry by the social worker, Tamara began to share her history. The fourth of five children, each fathered by a different man, she was removed from her mother's care at age 3 due to mother's severe depressive episodes and occasional neglect and physical abuse of the children. Tamara was placed subsequently with her favorite aunt, but this arrangement was short-lived. Although the aunt loved and wanted to keep her, the demands of raising her own children and her work responsibilities made caring for another child too difficult. Tamara was placed in the first of several foster homes and, over time, lost contact with her siblings. Another stable figure of her early life, her beloved grandmother, died suddenly at the time Tamara was placed in care.

Tamara's aunt visited her in her first foster home frequently. A few months after the placement began, she noticed that Tamara was acting strangely. Typically a chatterbox, she seemed withdrawn, preoccupied, and cried over seemingly minor incidents. The foster mother reported that Tamara had begun to wet her bed and was periodically encopretic. The aunt arranged for a physical examination, during which the pediatrician detected bruising around Tamara's genitals. This finding led to an investigation that revealed Tamara had been sexually abused by one of the foster parents' adolescent sons. Tamara was returned briefly to her aunt's home, but by age 6 she was placed in foster care again.

Despite this turbulent early history, Tamara did well in grade school. Teachers did remark that she daydreamed, appeared depressed periodically, and kept to herself on the playground. At puberty, she began skipping school and staying out past her curfew. She became pregnant at 15 and, subsequent to an abortion arranged by her aunt, she became despondent and acted out more. At 16 she "fell in love" with a boy whom she believed would stay with her forever. When she became pregnant again, however, he rejected her. This time she was determined to keep her baby: Finally she would have someone who would fill the emotional void left in the wake of all her losses and failed attachments.

Although Tamara recounted this story with little affect, the social worker was deeply moved listening to it. When Tamara described her fantasies that, at last, this baby would make her happy, the worker commented, "Now I think I understand why you named her Hope." Tamara looked directly into the worker's eyes, nodded somberly, and, for the first time, tears rolled down her cheeks. The worker marked this as a key affective moment in their work—Tamara had admitted her further into her inner world.

Just before their next scheduled meeting, however, Tamara phoned the worker to say she was feeling terrible and did not want to meet. She said she'd been staying in bed the last couple of days and hadn't cleaned the apartment. The worker asked Tamara if she thought what they had talked about in the previous meeting had upset her, and Tamara said she'd been crying since, missing Hope terribly. The worker said, "You know, Tamara, I'm going to come over anyway. If you decide once I'm there that you still prefer not to meet, that's okay. But I have a feeling it might help to talk more about all this." When the worker arrived, Tamara looked drawn and tired but said it would be fine it the worker stayed, so she sat quietly with

Tamara a while. As she was leaving, Tamara said, "Wait—I want to show you something. She unfolded a letter her favorite aunt had written to her when she entered foster care. The letter expressed the aunt's pride in Tamara, encouraged her to be a "good girl," and concluded with "never forget that I love you." Tamara wept as she read this letter aloud to the worker, the worker's own eyes tearing as well. They scheduled another appointment 2 days later, with the worker feeling that Tamara seemed ready to continue her story.

Tamara had quit school when Hope was born and became a very devoted and capable mother. Fortunately, her foster family agreed to incorporate Hope until Tamara "aged out" of the foster care system at age 18. During this period, Tamara acquired her GED and got a part-time job. Things apparently were going along well until Hope reached about 18 months. As a lively, confident, assertive toddler, Hope began to want to do things her own way. Tamara found herself getting increasingly irritated with Hope's feisty "attitude," began yelling more, and, to her horror, hit Hope several times. She tried to control her escalating anger but found herself "going off" on Hope more and more often. Her experience of these episodes was that she would become suddenly "not myself," almost as though she were watching someone else. Sometimes she couldn't recall exactly what had happened but would later "come to" and feel dreadful remorse. One day when Hope was running through the apartment, she tripped over a lamp cord, and the lamp fell and broke. Raging, Hope picked up the base of the lamp and slammed it into Hope, thus breaking her arm. Horrified, she knew Hope required medical attention, and, on the bus ride to the hospital, contrived the story she originally told the emergency room staff.

The evolution of this story took several months. The social worker's persistence in "staying with" Tamara seemed to make it safe enough for Tamara to let herself be known. With each revelation, there was some retreat from the relationship on Tamara's part, but repairing these disruptions became easier as the months went by. The worker helped Tamara tie her puzzling, unwanted feelings and behavior to her many past losses and attachment disruptions, and was able to interpret her emotional retreats from the worker in these terms as well. As she gained more insight into

the origins of her abusive behavior, Tamara's narrative became more coherent, and her affect more closely matched the content of her story.
Over time, she agreed to enroll in one of the agency's parenting classes
and joined a support group for women whose children were in foster care
and for whom reunification was likely. The worker helped Tamara find
employment that included a job-training component. Ultimately reunification was achieved, and periodic contacts with Tamara over ensuing
years indicated that Hope was flourishing in school and that her development was proceeding apace.

PSYCHONEUROBIOLOGICAL SUBSTRATE
OF CHILD WELFARE CASE

Tamara's social worker had received training at her agency in the psychoneurobiology of early trauma and its sequelae in attachment vulnerabilities. From her work experience with clients whose attachment histories
were often characterized by multiple losses and various types of trauma,
she approached her cases with awareness that, without intervention,
these histories tended to repeat themselves across generations. Drawn
especially to object relations theory, she believed that the establishment
of a therapeutic holding environment (Winnicott, 1965d) was essential to
the success of any intervention, and she understood that establishing such
an environment was a formidable challenge when clients' early caregiving
environments had not "held" them in contexts of safety, continuity, and
predictability.

The social worker in this case did not know at first that Hope's mother
had come from a traumatic background. Despite considerable evidence
that abusing caregivers have often been abused, she was aware that this
was not always the case. She approached Tamara with an attitude of re-
spectful inquiry that emphasized the social work effort to individualize
each client rather than imposing preconceived ideas about her history.
Nevertheless, the social worker's experience with similar cases suggested
to her that Hope's injury was likely the result of abuse. This hypothesis
was strengthened for her when Tamara, although fiercely protesting at
first, did not put up more resistance to the CYS investigation and Hope's

placement. Moreover, the guarded and adversarial posture Tamara assumed in the initial phase of the intervention suggested a history of past experiences that had led her to be wary and distrustful of those professing to be "helpful."

Setting aside any urgency to getting Tamara to "confess" the abuse or to reveal details of her situation and its history, the social worker made establishing a relationship her first priority. In preparation, she tuned into feelings and fantasies she became aware of, as a result of the nurse practitioner's warning that Tamara was "hell on wheels." Her mental images of an angry, demanding young woman generated some anxiety, but she regulated her level of anxiety by reflectively considering that Tamara, too, was likely anxious about meeting a stranger—a stranger with authority. Being "hell on wheels" could be a behavioral defense against feelings of shame, humiliation, and helplessness. This capacity to "mentalize" (Fonagy et al., 2002) about Tamara's possible state of mind enhanced the social worker's empathy for Tamara and helped her keep a calm, steady, and open approach when she met her.

Early in the intervention, the social worker paid close attention to Tamara's tolerance for physical closeness and constructed the "space" between them accordingly, employing such maneuvers as moving from the emergency room cubicle to the cafeteria. Also, sensing that a too-arousing affective approach would heighten Tamara's anxiety, the worker titrated her own typically lively, enthusiastic affect in order to attune it more closely to Tamara's affective expressions.

When Tamara struck out angrily at the worker in response to learning about the need to place Hope in temporary foster care, the worker felt frightened and experienced some physical symptoms of anxiety. Schore (2003b) suggested that an important qualification for clinicians working with affect-dysregulated clients is a capacity to become aware of their own right-hemispherically generated, visceral somatic countertransference reactions to the client's transferential affects. By activating her own abilities to organize and reflect upon these countertransference reactions as probable cues to Tamara's sense of feeling shamed, frightened, and attacked, the worker was able to respond empathically to Tamara's anger and sustain enough engagement to arrange a second meeting.

When Tamara failed to appear for this meeting, the worker knew it was crucial to telephone her to demonstrate that she was keeping her in mind. The worker was not surprised that Tamara didn't come for the meeting and mused that she was calibrating the pace of the relationship according to what she could tolerate. The worker's subsequent observation of Tamara's playful engagement with Hope in the hospital and Hope's animated response suggested that pre-attachment bonding had probably gone well between the two and that, if Tamara had abused Hope, it might have been recent and more episodic than chronic. This hypothesis gained some affirmation when the pediatric and neurological examination of Hope revealed that her development was generally within normal limits and that she related without fear to hospital staff.

After Hope's discharge to foster care, the worker arranged to continue meeting with Tamara at her apartment, negating Tamara's expectations that she would be transferred to another worker. As Beebe and Lachmann (2002) suggested, such relational "surprises" tend to solidify continuity in relationships with people whose earlier histories have been characterized by discontinuity and disruption. Noting Tamara's willingness to have the worker visit her home, the social worker felt more optimistic about developing a strong working alliance. This optimism left her unprepared, therefore, for the strength of her negative reactions when Tamara was absent for the first home visit. These reactions had an urgent, visceral quality, but rather than processing these affects reflectively as before, the worker acted them out by calling Tamara and discharging her anger inappropriately.

Later, her reflective capacity restored, the social worker could conceptualize what had happened as a mutually constructed enactment secondary to projective identification that was likely based on simultaneous activation of the pair's attachment-related neural networks (Greatrex, 2002). Tamara's behavior had communicated to the social worker what it felt like to be dismissed and left alone, and had also served the unconscious purpose of finding out how trustworthy and accepting the worker could be. As Westen and Gabbard suggested, clinicians, like everyone else, "differ in the extent to which their temperament and experience have laid down strong neural 'tracks' that predispose them to take on particular roles, such as to become a shaming object under certain circumstances" (2002, p. 118). Tamara's rejecting behavior touched a vulnerability in the worker that led to her retaliation, thus confirming Tamara's expectation that the worker could not tolerate and accept her affects and behavior.

Following this enactment, the worker moved quickly to repair the relational disruption (Beebe & Lachmann, 2002). Her apology seemed to rerail their tenuous connection. During the next visit, when Tamara was still wary and looked more at the TV than at the worker, the worker mused that the TV was serving as a buffer for Tamara, whose discomfort with closeness needed to be diluted by an intermediary object. In a later visit, when the worker became aware of an urge to "give up" on Tamara, she was able to use her impulse more productively as a signal of projective identification. Because Tamara had not yet begun to verbalize any discomfort, the worker used her own feelings to interpret to Tamara her hunch that Tamara expected the worker to give up on her, as others may have. Such interventions gradually solidified the working alliance, and the social worker believed she and Tamara were slowly establishing a pattern of ongoing regulation (Beebe & Lachmann, 2002). As Tamara began to tell her story, the social worker's earlier hypothesis that Tamara herself had suffered early abuse appeared to be confirmed.

The social worker's knowledge of the neurological effects of trauma helped her appreciate that some of the traumata in her clients' lives are too overwhelming to be processed cognitively and that, for young children in her caseload, immature cognitive development would make such processing impossible. As a result, such trauma is stored, unprocessed, in implicit negative affective memory (Bromberg, 2003) and is less likely to be verbalized than somatized or acted out. Either because of early trauma-induced hippocampal damage or as a result of later trauma so overwhelming to cognitive capacities that it bypasses the memory-processing hippocampus altogether, neural networks of implicit and explicit memory remain unintegrated.

Given the history of Tamara's multiple losses during her early years—and the likelihood that no one acknowledged her pain or helped her talk about these losses—the social worker was surprised that her attachment

style was not of the disorganized/disoriented type. Fonagy (1998) reported
that such early unmourned loss often eventuates in this insecure attachment type. Rather, Tamara's attachment style seemed to be primarily
avoidant. Needing to cope with so many comings and goings of caregivers led her to avoid becoming too attached to anyone. This formulation could explain her initial wariness and hostility toward the social
worker. Yet Tamara had formed a strong attachment to Hope and was
slowly beginning to allow herself to get closer to the social worker. This
willingness suggested to the worker that Tamara had gleaned enough from
her relationships with her mother, grandmother, and aunt to sustain hope
that a close, nurturing relationship was possible.

Severe trauma entered Tamara's life when she left her aunt's home.
The traumatic effects of her sexual abuse in the first foster home led to
symptoms that prompted Tamara's aunt to seek professional help. Hearing
this story, the social worker believed it likely that Tamara's preoccupation
and daydreaming in school were forms of mild dissociation. Dissociation
has been described as a form of hypnoid autoregulation during which
conscious awareness of an affectively overwhelming event is detached
from emotional and physiological processing. This unconscious defensive
maneuver enables the traumatized person to escape the immediacy of the
abusive situation. The worker hypothesized that Tamara had relied on dissociation to endure her abuse; a hypothesis that was strengthened by her
description of breaking Hope's arm. Her descriptions of "going off," becoming "not myself," and "coming to" without recalling what had happened suggested that Tamara's abuse of Hope occurred during a transient
dissociative episode triggered by dysregulated affect.

During early episodes of abuse and dissociation, the brain's information-
processing capacities become disorganized. Both top–down and right–left
processing are interrupted, leaving the victim of abuse awash in dysregulated affect. Severe trauma also sets off a neurochemical cascade of neurotransmitter and hormonal changes that can permanently compromise
aspects of neural integration. A marked increase in norephinephrine triggers anxiety, arousal, and the automatic, amygdala-based fight-or-flight
response to feeling threatened. Increased dopamine results in withdrawal
and perceptual distortions, and increases in endogenous opioids induce

dissociation that impairs reality testing. A decrease in serotonin can predispose the traumatized individual to depression, anxiety, irritability, aggression, and violence (Cozolino, 2002).

Memory is also negatively influenced by trauma. Stress-induced increases in glucocorticoid levels can, by inducing neuronal overpruning and cell death, result in reduced hippocampal volume with subsequent deficits in explicit memory capacities. Importantly, findings from neuroimaging studies have suggested that this volume is reduced more in the cognitive, linguistically and positively biased left hemisphere than in the affective, negatively biased right (Teicher, 2002). By inference, this hippocampal volume difference would make it difficult for victims of abuse to retrieve positive memories of soothing interactions when overwhelmed by negative affects. As a result, individuals may be left with physiological and affective "memories" of trauma but are unable to attenuate them by placing them in context or activating integrative processes of cortical appraisal and regulation. Situations subsequently appraised as threatening or anger producing set off trauma-imprinted "low road" amygdala–hippocampus neural pathways that bypass the "high road" contextualizing, reality-testing capacities of the orbitofrontal cortex (Cozolino, 2002; LeDoux, 1996; Schore, 2003a).

We can surmise that, in Tamara's case, her striking out at Hope was a result of such dissociated, automatic, and neurally unintegrated impulses. She seemed to do well with Hope during her early infancy, until age 2. When Hope began to show developmentally normal signs of separating and assertively exploring the world beyond Tamara, this behavior may have reawakened Tamara's implicit memories of her early losses. Because Tamara had been abused, the aggressive impulses aroused by her perception of Hope's behavior as rejecting induced amygdala-based unprocessed aggressive arousal—Panksepp's (1998) rage command system. Experiencing Hope's destruction of the lamp as a personal attack, Tamara seems to have dissociated while her "fight" mode overtook her. Schore (2003a), referencing research by Wheeler, Davidson, and Tomarken (1993), concluded that such overwhelming impulses are believed to be the result of extreme levels of right orbitofrontal subcortical activation. Individuals thus aroused "are thought to exhibit a negative affective response to a very low-intensity negative affect elicitor, and to be impaired in the ability to terminate a negative emotion once it has begun" (Schore, 2003a, 224).

Over the many months that the social worker saw Tamara intensively, and as Tamara became more comfortable talking about her childhood, the worker provided psychoeducation about how early relational traumatic stress can lead to "losing track" of rational thought while feelings take over. Such interventions helped Tamara feel less shamed by what she had done and more comfortable sharing her story. Initially Tamara's recounting of her life was fragmented and disorganized. At points when Tamara seemed at a loss for words, the social worker used her own subjective experience to "muse" about Tamara's state of mind, thus modeling the reflective function. She also asked questions to clarify for herself, and to organize for Tamara, the disjointed narrative. From a neurobiological perspective, the social worker's efforts to help Tamara put the bits and pieces of her story into a coherent narrative helped her develop more integrative and efficient top–down and right–left neural processing. As noted earlier, such increases in neural network integration promote more effective affect regulation (Cozolino, 2002).

The level of attachment between Tamara and the social worker was strengthened by the occurrence of positive heightened affective moments (Beebe & Lachmann, 2002). One of these occurred when the social worker expressed her understanding of the reason Tamara had named her daughter *Hope*. This interpretive remark moved Tamara to tears and must have given her the experience of being empathically "heard" and understood. Another episode was initiated by Tamara, who shared with the worker the letter her aunt had written when releasing her to foster care. Such moments could be seen as facilitating a mourning process that helped Tamara access the sadness and grief that she had long covered up by a "false self" adversarial posture. Hope did give Tamara another chance for attachment, but it was conditional on Hope's remaining symbiotically close to her. When Hope violated this condition by beginning to separate and challenge her mother's limits, Tamara once again felt rejected and abandoned. Her current feelings tapped implicit memories of the rage she felt, both about her multiple losses and the sexual abuse. Because the memories were implicit, they could only be experienced unconsciously and acted out. In talking through Tamara's feelings in partnership with her, the social worker attempted to help her transpose them from subsymbolic to symbolic form, thus rendering them more amendable to conscious control.

Finally, the social worker augmented her own therapeutic efforts with additional psychoeducation in the form of a parenting group. Also, in referring Tamara to a group where she would hear the stories of women in similar circumstances, the worker hoped to help further strengthen her relational holding environment while providing a context in which she could feel less shamed. Throughout the intervention, the social worker remained aware that, in addition to the early relational trauma in Tamara's life, she experienced the chronic, day-to-day stress of poverty, life in an urban public housing project, and racial discrimination. These sociostructural factors also challenge people's capacity for affect regulation. The worker acted as an advocate for Tamara in helping her find employment with opportunities for further training and advancement.

Together, all the worker's interventions provided Tamara with the experience of a positive attachment relationship with a "new" object. Better prepared to regulate her affects, and with a broadened, more nuanced affective repertoire, Tamara was helped to support and respond adaptively to Hope's development in ways that held the promise of interrupting the cycle of intergenerational relational trauma.

The following case study illustrates the use of a cognitive–behavioral approach with a client presenting with an anxiety disorder. Here new findings about the neurobiology of fear inform the social worker's assessment and intervention. The inclusion of relationship-building processes in the treatment reflects today's increasing emphasis on the interpersonal dimensions of cognitive–behavioral work.

ELLEN: A CASE FROM A COMMUNITY MENTAL HEALTH CENTER

On opening the door of the waiting room at the community mental health center to meet his new clients, the social worker saw two women sitting side by side. One of them appeared terror-stricken; the other looked irritated. Introducing himself, the social worker invited the pair into his office and noticed that Ellen, the one who appeared frightened, moved her chair as far as possible from his. Automatically, the worker moved his chair a bit closer and leaned forward. This action seemed to startle Ellen, who quickly leaned further back in her chair. Sensing Ellen's discomfort, the worker moved his chair back to its original position and leaned back as well.

Meanwhile, the other client, Marianne, appeared comfortable, if impatient, in her chair nearer the worker. When the worker asked the women what had brought them to his office, Ellen turned to Marianne expectantly, signaling her to explain. With a sigh, Marianne began. It became clear that the pair, both in their late 20s and partners for 7 years, had recently structured their lives around Ellen's inability to leave the house. Her agoraphobia had begun about 3 months ago. Standing in line at the post office, Ellen was suddenly overcome by panic. She began to perspire and gasp for air, her heart pounding, "for no reason." Feeling she was going to faint, she raced outside where, shortly, she began to calm down.

More comfortable now that Marianne had begun, Ellen tentatively began to describe her situation in more detail. She thought the first panic episode was a fluke and returned to the post office a day or 2 later with no problem. But a week later, again standing in a post office line, her symptoms reappeared in full force. This time she began to believe she might have a heart attack, die, or go crazy, and again she fled the building. Although less acute, a similar reaction in the post office a few days later cemented her decision not to return. Ellen thought avoiding the post office would solve a circumscribed problem until she had a full-blown attack standing in line at the supermarket. Sure she was dying, she left her cart and, sobbing, ran outside to her car. Lines of people anywhere—the movies, the supermarket, concerts—became triggers for Ellen, and she began avoiding them.

Although puzzled about Ellen's difficulties, Marianne was sympathetic and tried to accommodate her needs to avoid the triggering situations. Both were flabbergasted, however, when, on a Sunday afternoon walk in their quiet suburban neighborhood, Ellen's panic returned. She ran back to the house, certain that she would die if she did not reach safety there. Because her symptoms were happening in so many situations, she became convinced she was having mild heart attacks. But a checkup by a cardiologist, as well as a complete physical, revealed no organic basis for her distress.

Gradually, Ellen began to find ways to stay in the house to avoid further episodes. She arranged with the group of doctors for whom she transcribed medical records to work from her computer at home and e-mail her reports. Because Marianne worked as a paralegal in a building only a few blocks away, it was easy for her to run errands during her lunch break or after work.

Knowing that panic attacks often commence during a period of unusual stress, the worker was not surprised to learn that Ellen's had begun shortly after Marianne had been offered a better job in the city, 45 miles from their home. On hearing Marianne's news, Ellen tried to be enthusiastic; but she could not ignore an immediate sense of apprehension at the prospect of Marianne being so far away. To Ellen, this felt like the first separation in their relationship, and she realized that, over the years, she had gained a degree of emotional comfort from knowing that Marianne's office was nearby. She shared her concerns with Marianne, and several discussions about her worries had increased the tension in the relationship. Finally, Ellen asked Marianne to turn down the promotion "if you really love me." For Marianne, this was the last straw—she declared that she would accept the position and that Ellen had to "grow up" and pull herself together if they were to remain a couple.

It was after this confrontation that Marianne convinced Ellen to make an appointment at the agency, known in the community to have a program specifically focused on the treatment of anxiety disorders. Leaving the house to keep their appointment took every ounce of courage Ellen could muster. She had a panic attack in the car on the way and was still highly agitated when the social worker stepped into the waiting room.

After two appointments during which he gathered some basic information, the social worker began the intervention by seeing the couple together a few times to educate them about the psychophysiology of anxiety and panic. He explained aspects of the neurophysiology of the fear response, pointing out that Ellen's automatic and overwhelming attacks suggested that her capacity to think through and regulate her anxiety was being inhibited by the strength of her raw fear and her impulses to flee. He pointed out that the attacks are not life threatening, nor are they signs of impending insanity. He described the typical course of such attacks, emphasizing that they usually last 3–10 minutes and only rarely more than 30 minutes (Maxmen & Ward, 1995). This psychoeducation seemed to relieve Ellen somewhat and helped Marianne be less impatient with her. At this point, the social worker began to meet with Ellen alone, with the understanding that Marianne would join them periodically. He acknowledged Marianne for being patient and supportive of Ellen, and he also pointed out that, by standing her ground about her new job and suggesting therapy, Marianne was making it possible for Ellen to address her difficulties directly.

The agency's cognitive–behavioral approach to anxiety disorders was based on a conceptualization of such disorders as expressions of affect dysregulation. Included in this conceptualization is an appreciation for the neurological elements in such dysregulation. In the specific case of panic disorder with agoraphobia, agency clinicians began their intervention with home visits. This strategy both respected the degree of fear experienced by people with these symptoms and provided the opportunity to begin to forge a therapeutic alliance in the setting in which clients felt safest. Once the alliance was strong enough, clients, with the active support of the clinician as "coach," were gradually and incrementally exposed to the situations that acted as triggers for their attacks. While engaged in this "travel work," clients were asked to verbalize the feelings and thoughts accompanying their exposure to the feared situations.

Before initiating such an intervention with Ellen, the social worker used the first of several home visits to learn more about her history and to begin to develop a one-to-one relationship with her. He realized that, without the backdrop of a supportive, empathic relationship that helped Ellen feel emotionally safe, the cognitive–behavioral component of the intervention was unlikely to succeed.

During their first meeting without Marianne, Ellen's anxiety, so apparent in the first meeting but having abated in subsequent couple sessions, reappeared. She again seemed frightened and agitated, her eyes darting apprehensively around the living room. When the social worker commented that Marianne's absence seemed to be hard for her, Ellen nodded slowly and became tearful. She was quiet for several minutes, and the social worker did not intrude. When it felt right to him, he asked Ellen if she could talk a bit about what she was feeling during the silence. As she haltingly described her feelings of fear and a sense of disorientation, the social worker nodded, made occasional nonverbal utterances, but spoke little. By their third session, an observer of the pair might have noted that the social worker's facial expressions were often similar to Ellen's and that the manner in which they were sitting in their respective chairs was remarkably similar. This facial mirroring and postural sharing were outside the awareness of either partner in the therapeutic couple and suggested the beginning establishment of ongoing mutual regulation.

As their relationship developed, the social worker encouraged Ellen to describe her history in more detail. He learned that her mother recalled her being shy, easily upset, and inhibited from toddlerhood on. She seemed equally attached to both parents and enjoyed especially her father's attentions. She had difficulty separating from home to begin school, and for the first few years her mother picked her up each day to bring her home for lunch. As Ellen's story developed, the social worker began to hypothesize that her mother may have benefited from Ellen's temperamental disposition. Given his knowledge that anxiety disorders often run in families, he was not surprised to learn that Ellen's mother had several phobias. Ellen also described her maternal grandmother as a virtual recluse by the time she was 40, suggesting the likelihood that she was agoraphobic.

The parents divorced when Ellen was 4 years old, and it appeared that her mother may have turned to her to assuage her own anxieties about separation. The divorce was acrimonious, and Ellen's father soon took employment in another state. She saw him only rarely after that. Ellen and her mother became a close twosome, and Ellen always had the feeling that her mother depended on her to make her happy.

Ellen's closeness to her mother continued through middle childhood, but with adolescence, she began to pull away, and their relationship grew more conflicted. Ellen's efforts to separate and explore her social world led to frequent arguments. Invariably, however, Ellen would feel so guilty about her anger that she would put her own needs on hold in order to pacify her mother's need to keep her nearby. This pattern changed when Ellen met Marianne in her early 20s. Ellen's mother was distraught when the couple moved in together, but this time Ellen was able to tolerate her guilt about leaving her.

During her account of her history to the social worker, Ellen became aware that she blamed her mother for the divorce, thus robbing her of her adored father. As they explored her feelings about this, Ellen suddenly recalled that she and her mother had had a heated argument during a telephone call about 2 hours before her first panic attack. Ellen remembered worrying after the call that she may have alienated her mother permanently with some of her angry remarks.

By the second month of treatment, when the working alliance was on solid footing, Ellen and the social worker devised a strategy designed to help Ellen begin to leave the house and return to the situations that triggered her panic attacks. They began with small steps. At first, Ellen was asked to walk to the sidewalk in front of the house with the worker at her side. When Ellen could do this with some degree of comfort, the worker remained on the porch, offering calm encouragement. Later, they applied this strategy to helping Ellen walk to the end of her street, thereby slowly increasing Ellen's tolerance for leaving "home base." At first, Ellen's anxiety would escalate, and she would freeze in place and hyperventilate. At these points the social worker would match the pace of his breathing to Ellen's, then, making eye contact, would gradually slow his own breathing. Invariably, Ellen's breathing would slow in tandem with the worker's and she would begin to feel calmer.

Other behavioral techniques were also employed to assist Ellen in managing the level of her anxiety during exposure episodes. The social worker helped her construct an "anxiety scale," with 0 as "no anxiety" and 10 as "maximum anxiety." With this tool, Ellen could better objectify and calibrate her anxiety level in a manner that gave her some sense of control In various fear-arousing situations, she could say to herself, "This is a 6" or "This is almost a 10." When, over time, this self-monitoring method revealed a decrease in the scale levels, she could see objective evidence of improvement. This tool was augmented by instruction in deep breathing and other methods of relaxation training.

Cognitive methods also assisted Ellen in tolerating the exposure exercises. In exploring Ellen's "self-talk" as she became panicky, the worker learned that Ellen was saying to herself, "I'm going to die from a heart attack or stroke! I'm going to suffocate here—I have to get out!" Reminding Ellen that panic attacks are not life threatening and that they typically abate in a few minutes, he suggested that she change her self talk to "This too shall pass."

Over several months, the pair ventured further and further away from Ellen's home and toward the original panic-inducing situations. They visited the supermarket, the worker at Ellen's side talking her through her anxiety and coaching her to employ the anxiety-reducing tools she'd learned. During the most affectively intensive exposure exercises, the social worker encouraged her to talk about the feelings that were aroused. Had she ever had these feelings in the past? In what situations? Was she alone? If not, who was there with her? What was happening? In one notable episode during a walk in an open park that Ellen had been avoiding, she began shaking uncontrollably, burst into tears, and sobbed for several minutes. With the worker's calm encouragement, she talked about how much she missed her father and raged at her mother for never acknowledging her grief. The worker's knowledge that the psychodynamic aspects of panic attacks can often be traced to unresolved grief helped him understand, and interpret to Ellen, the meaning of her outburst. Her sense of "losing" Marianne had stirred her previously repressed grief over a loss she had never completely mourned.

Similarly moving affective episodes and the worker's interpretive work equipped Ellen with increased insight about the etiology of her difficulties. Together, such insight-oriented processes and the cognitive–behavioral interventions helped Ellen gain increasing control over her anxiety. Gradually, she became more confident in her ability to confront the feared situations, culminating in her successful negotiation of a long line in the post office. Returning to the car where the worker was waiting, she was excited to report that she accomplished this goal while mentally marking only a "3" on her anxiety scale. Finally, she was able to drive alone and celebrated this accomplishment by meeting Marianne for lunch and announcing that she no longer required her services as a chauffeur.

PSYCHONEUROBIOLOGICAL SUBSTRATE OF PANIC DISORDER CASE

Although assessing Ellen's difficulties as comprising a classic case of panic disorder with agoraphobia, and therefore concluding that a primarily cognitive–behavioral approach would be most helpful, the social worker began the intervention by focusing on establishing a relational context of therapeutic safety. From the first contact, he carefully observed Ellen's expressions of anxiety and shaped his own responses in accordance with her comfort level. In the initial interview, for example, Ellen evinced a kind of startle reaction to the worker's moving his chair closer to her and leaning forward. Although not completely conscious of his response, the worker intuitively adjusted his own posture to give Ellen more physical space. In their first one-to-one session Ellen's acute anxiety reappeared. This time, the worker attempted to give words to what she might be feeling in Marianne's absence, a strategy that elicited tearful affect and appeared to help her feel less frightened. The worker's approach was consistent with the current trend toward integrating attention to interpersonal dynamics into cognitive–behavioral approaches (Bradley, 2000).

Throughout the assessment and intervention phases, the social worker drew on his knowledge of the biopsychosocial determinants of anxiety disorders. There appeared to be a history of these disorders in her maternal lineage, suggesting the likelihood of a biological predisposition in Ellen's case. Most studies find that 30–50% of the variance in these disorders is explained by genetic factors (Bradley, 2000). These factors appear to render some individuals more vulnerable than others to environmental stressors.

Efforts to relate anxiety disorders to constitutional and temperamental differences identify three common traits: neuroticism, emotionality, and inhibition. Those with high degrees of neuroticism have a highly reactive limbic system that generates high levels of arousal in the autonomic nervous system long after an anxiety-provoking stimulus has ended. Many have elevated levels of emotionality, a component of which is fearfulness, that appears to be inherited and related to temperament. Finally, the trait of inhibition, expressed in a tendency of individuals to be slower to explore and more likely to retreat from unfamiliar situations, appears to be strongly associated with inborn temperament. Together, these traits suggest that anxiety secondary to stress reactivity includes components of heritability and constitutional predisposition. Their neurobiological basis involves limbic system structures such as the amygdala and the hippocampus and their interconnections (Bradley, 2000).

Anxiety is related to the affect of fear and is connected to the core biological fight-or-flight mechanisms that have served the purpose of evolutionary survival. As noted in Chapter 4, the fear system is located in the nuclei of the amygdala and is expressed typically in avoidance, "freezing," or fleeing the feared situation. These responses, which are results of activation of the *fear* command system, are accompanied by increased heart rate, hyperventilation, and a redistribution of blood flow to skeletal muscles (Panksepp, 1998).

Neuroscientists believe that some circumscribed fears, such as the fear of snakes, spiders, closed spaces, or heights, appear to be specific to primates and have become hard-wired during evolution in order to foster the goal of basic survival. With human evolution, the amygdala has been expanded to accommodate increasingly complex and sophisticated cognitive, sensory, and affective processes associated with the appraisal of potentially fearsome situations. In addition, human amygdaloid circuitry interacts with the most evolved areas of the cerebral cortex. As a result, primitive fear responses designed for survival are combined with the sophisticated cognitive processes, including the capacity for fantasy and imagination. This developmental advance means that we can become anxious about situations that, to outside observers, appear irrational (Cozolino, 2002).

One of the most clinically applicable conceptualizations of the neurobiology of anxiety is LeDoux's (1996) description of the two neural pathways by which perception of a feared stimulus reaches the amygdala. As detailed in Chapter 3, LeDoux discovered that one pathway, termed the "low road," leads directly from the sense organs through the thalamus to the amygdala. Information moves along this pathway rapidly and reflexively. The amygdala immediately appraises the sensory input (from eyes, ears, nose, etc.) and translates it into fight-or-flight–based bodily reactions. This quick transmission signals the individual to respond to the fear-arousing stimulus before full awareness of what it is. (Recall LeDoux's example of a person coming upon a poisonous snake in the woods.) The fear system is put on high alert status with attendant physiological arousal.

The perceptual information also moves along the "high road," though at a slower pace, from the sensory organs to the thalamus, through circuits of the hippocampus and sensory cortex, and then to the amygdala. This pathway permits a more detailed and accurate representation of the stimulus. It is slower because it involves additional synaptic connections, compares the current stimulus to memories of similar situations, and facilitates conscious voluntary decision making about how to proceed (Cozolino, 2002). Assisted by the conscious executive functions of the cortical–hippocampal system, the brain is able to make a detailed appraisal of the stimulus and assign it meaning. In clinical work with anxiety, one goal of intervention is to use the conscious linguistic structures of the high road to inhibit and render more manageable the reactive, unconscious, and preverbal appraisals of the low-road pathways.

The amygdala and hippocampus, although they interact in fear-producing episodes, organize different and potentially dissociated memory systems (Cozolino, 2002). Recall that the amygdala stores nonconscious implicit memory whereas the hippocampus stores conscious explicit memory. When hippocampal activation is inhibited, the amygdala can produce anxiety reactions in the absence of real danger. This phenomenon is the neurobiological basis for panic attacks—sensing stimuli that, for a given individual, are symbolic of an earlier encountered danger situation, the amygdala sets off autonomic fight-or-flight reactions such as elevated heart rate, hyperventilation, and other symptoms of outright fear. Once this occurs, the tendency of the amygdala to generalize leads to activation of panic reactions to an increasing number of situations.

Interestingly, this neurobiological explanation of the etiology of anxiety is consistent with Freud's (1926/1959) psychoanalytic formulation of signal anxiety. According to this formulation, signal anxiety institutes defenses designed to help the individual cope either with an objective danger or to keep painful or unacceptable impulses out of awareness. Toward the latter goal, much anxiety remains unconscious while the defenses support adaptive and relatively comfortable functioning. When signal anxiety fails or has never been adequately developed, anxiety can override ego functioning and leave the person in the type of fearful state seen in panic and other anxiety disorders. Another way to view the failure of signal anxiety is that the direct thalamus–amygdala low-road transmission of fear-inducing sensory information has bypassed the cortical high road, thus short-circuiting the "signal" of danger that could help the individual more realistically assess it and regulate affect accordingly.

Representing the psychological component of the biopsychosocial perspective, cognitive–behavioral and social learning formulations suggest that, once anxiety is aroused in certain situations, it becomes generalized to similar situations or those symbolizing the original fear-inducing situation. In other words, anxiety can become a conditioned response, as seems to have occurred in Ellen's situation.

Finally, the knowledge that initial panic attacks typically occur during a period of unusual stress (Maxmen & Ward, 1995) speaks to the social component of panic disorder. In Ellen's case, the prospect of Marianne's relocation appeared to be such a stressor. Ellen's mother's description of her early years suggests shyness and vulnerabilities related to separation–individuation (Mahler, Pine, & Bergman, 1975). In adolescence, Ellen appeared to make concerted efforts to address these early vulnerabilities. Blos (1967) has referred to adolescence as a "second individuation," during which individuals have an opportunity to rework and consolidate the early childhood separation–individuation process. Ellen appeared to have used this opportunity adaptively when she met and moved in with Marianne. Things went well until Marianne's job offer—an occurrence that, to Ellen, symbolized separation and reawakened her earlier anxiety, thus triggering her initial panic attack.

Employing an integrative approach emphasizing cognitive–behavioral theory, the social worker began his intervention with psychoeducation for both Ellen and Marianne about the psychophysiology of anxiety. Thereafter, the worker created a "safe emergency" (Cozolino, 2002) when he separated the couple and began to see Ellen alone. Although frightened at first, Ellen responded well to the worker's empathic approach to her distress. To gather information while solidifying a therapeutic alliance, the worker began by taking a comprehensive history. Emerging information enabled him to confirm his initial impressions of the problem and, in collaboration with Ellen, begin to formulate an intervention plan.

To build on the increased cortical processing activated by psychoeducation, the next step in the intervention was to expose Ellen to a gradually intensified series of safe emergencies designed to combine increased cortical processing (cognition) with the affects aroused by the exposure. The goal in such strategies is to permit low-road fear circuitry to blend with high-road cortical circuitry in order to achieve greater neural network integration. Relaxation training, coupled with such cognition-focused tools as the anxiety scale and revised self-talk during panic episodes, helped Ellen begin to achieve conscious control of her thoughts and feelings. Neuroscientists have suggested that such strategies also enhance left-hemispheric cortical processing while inhibiting and regulating both right-hemispheric and subcortical activation (Cozolino, 2002).

Ellen's capacity to undertake exposure to situations known to trigger her panic depended on the physical presence and emotional support of the social worker. Hypothesizing that a psychosocial aspect of her panic related to separation anxiety, he at first stayed by her side as she attempted the steps in their plan. As she became less frightened, he slowly retreated, allowing Ellen to gain more confidence in her capacity to regulate her fear autonomously. To further enhance cortical processing of her affects, he encouraged her to verbalize what she was thinking and feeling during episodes of exposure. The episode during which Ellen got in touch with the grief and rage associated with the loss of her father became a "heightened affective moment" (Beebe & Lachmann, 2002) that further strengthened the therapeutic relationship.

Beyond eliciting a broader range of affect, the effort to help Ellen narrate her distress was conceptualized as another technique to help her achieve more cognitive control over her overwhelming reactions. In addition, the worker's and Ellen's narrative coconstruction of the historical etiology of her difficulties enabled her to ascribe meaning to reactions that had previously baffled her. Together, all the components of the social worker's integrative approach helped Ellen better regulate her affect, modify negative thought patterns, and alter her behavior in the context of increased insight.

The final case study illustrates the manner in which a subsystem in the family can regulate uncomfortable affects by scapegoating another family member who, in turn, acts them out. Here several typical family-focused interventions are reconceptualized as efforts to foster affect tolerance, diminish the need for projection, and enhance neural network integration.

THE WILSONS: A CASE FROM A FAMILY SERVICE AGENCY

When Andrea Wilson telephoned the family service agency, she said that she and her husband, Michael, had "a mess on our hands." Asked to elaborate, she revealed that their 17-year-old son, Frank, had just been suspended from school after one of his teachers caught him smoking marijuana in the restroom. This infraction of school rules was the "last straw" for the principal, who had seen Frank in his office frequently over the last several months for truancy and fistfights with classmates. After meeting with Frank and making little headway in understanding or helping him modify his behavior, the school counselor phoned the Wilsons and referred them to the agency.

Because the agency typically employed a family systems approach in such situations, the social worker assigned to the case arranged for Frank and his parents to come in for the first interview together. Once they entered her office, the worker paid careful attention to where they chose to sit and how they interacted with each other. In addition to the worker's chair by her desk, there were three chairs grouped across from a couch in the office. Interestingly, Andrea and Michael took chairs at either end of the grouping, and Andrea motioned for Frank to take the one in between. Frank hesitated, looking at the couch for a moment, then, after giving Andrea an exasperated look, flopped down in the chair between his parents. Scooting down in his chair, his legs stretched out in front, Frank began flipping a cigarette lighter open and closed while gazing out the office window.

The worker began by asking the Wilsons what had brought them to the agency. Andrea and Michael looked at each other, each apparently waiting for the other to begin. Frank continued to look out the window. After a few awkward moments, the worker said, "Sometimes it's hard to begin." With this, Andrea declared, "I don't even know where to begin! We've had nothing but trouble with Frank this year—his junior year, when he's supposed to be looking at colleges. Now he tells us he's not *going* to college—he wants to "take a year off" and move into the city with some of his cronies! He's disrespectful to us, ignores the limits we try to set, and, if he's not out with his friends half the night, he holes himself up in this room, staying up till 2:00 or 3:00 in the morning. He does nothing to help around the house and refuses to carry on a conversation with us. I've just had it. And now this school thing!"

Michael remained quiet. When the worker asked what he thought was going on, he said, "I guess I just second everything she's said. I don't get as upset as she does, but Frank's getting to be a pain. We really don't know what to do anymore."

When the worker asked Frank for his view of the problem, he kept looking out the window and shrugged. After a few moments, Andrea said, "Well, go on! Tell her—we'd like to know, too!" Frank, glaring at his mother, muttered "Yeah, right." Andrea immediately jumped in: "See? This is what he *always* does. We never get a straight answer!" The worker asked her how not getting answers felt to her, and she said, "Well, it's like we don't exist. He used to be the nicest kid, and now he treats us like dirt." The worker noted that, asked how *she* felt, Andrea replied in terms of *we*.

Turning again to Frank, the worker said, "You know, there's no rule that you have to talk here; but it would help me get a better picture of why you and your parents are here. So far I only have their version." Almost a minute passed, and the parents looked increasingly uncomfortable. Finally, Frank declared, "Look, this is all their idea. I don't know why the hell I'm even here! They get all bent out of shape because I stay out late sometimes. They *never* let me take the car. If it was up to them, I'd be a prisoner in that house. And staying in with them isn't exactly a picnic. *She* has this fantasy that we should be like the Bradys or something."

Andrea, who'd been barely containing herself, interjected, "That's just not fair! It isn't like that at all!" Gently but firmly, the worker said that if they were to begin to address the problems that have brought them to the agency, they needed to establish a rule for how they would communicate: she suggested that when one person is talking, others should wait until he or she is finished before responding. Andrea said, "But what if . . ."—to which the worker said, "Okay, I know this is a hard rule, but trust me, we'll all understand this better if each person has a chance to speak uninterrupted."

The worker asked Frank if he had anything else to say. He shook his head "no" and slid further down in his chair. The worker then turned to Andrea and asked her to summarize what she had heard Frank say. "Well, I guess he feels like a prisoner." Turning to Frank, she declared, "We think we've made a pretty comfortable life for you. A prisoner, ha!" The worker said to Andrea, "I guess this is another kind of communication rule—you'll find that I'll frequently ask each of you to feed back what you heard others say. It's a way to make sure everybody is heard. The rule is to just feed back what you hear without adding commentary. Can you agree to that?" Andrea, looking miffed, waited a moment before nodding her head. The worker continued, "So, anything else you heard him say?" Andrea replied, "Well, he said we're not fun to be around." The worker exclaimed, "Good! That's the idea!"

The social worker then asked Michael what he had heard Frank say. He was quiet a moment, then said, "I guess he feels hemmed in, that he'd like the car more. But, jeez, he had it twice last week!" The worker said, "Again, try to feed back only what you heard him say." Frank replied, "Well, he feels like we're trying to be the Bradys and we're too strict." The worker said, "Okay, that's good. Now, did your parents seem to summarize what you said pretty well?" Frank grudgingly mumbled, "I guess."

The remainder of the session continued in this general pattern. Andrea was the most vocal of the three and, as before, Michael seemed to echo her ideas rather than add any of his own. The social worker was encouraged that Frank, though mostly silent, did make a few comments. The social worker scheduled another family meeting. Initially Frank bristled and said, "No way!" But again, the worker said she did not think it was fair to get only his parents' side of the story, and he reluctantly agreed to another appointment. The worker told the family that, for the next meeting, she would like to develop a family genogram—a three-generational genealogical diagram or "map" of the family (McGoldrick & Gerson, 1989).

The social worker viewed the genogram as a method to collect important family history and as a way to join the family system around a project. She saw this joining process as key to building a therapeutic working relationship with the family. In addition, seeing that the Wilsons were a family having trouble managing strong affects, she hoped to employ the genogram as a way to help them take some distance from the affective "heat" of their conflict by working with her on a more cognitively oriented task.

During construction and discussion of the genogram over the next two family sessions, the social worker learned that Frank was the youngest of five children, 5 years younger than his next oldest sibling. Frank had been a "surprise baby" who was born when Andrea and Michael were 35. Andrea reported being "thrilled" to learn she was pregnant again—"I love babies! It's what I do best!" She had been feeling a little sad since her 4-year-old had entered nursery school and was glad to have "a replacement baby." When asked what it was like for Frank to hear this story, he rolled his eyes and mumbled, "Sounds like some bad TV movie."

The first of the children had been born barely a year after Andrea and Michael married, in their early 20s, and the others came along at 2- or 3-year intervals. Andrea crowed proudly about the accomplishments of her first four children, the last of whom had moved out 6 months before the family had come to the agency. The couple's frugality and careful planning had made it possible for all four to finish college, while reserving enough funds to help Frank as well. Neither Andrea nor Michael had gone to college, and they were determined that their children would do so. This goal often strained their budget, given Michael's modest salary from his position as a postal worker and Andrea's small remuneration from her part-time work at a dress shop in their small rural community. Now in their 50s, they seemed deservingly proud of this accomplishment and were hurt and angry at Frank's declaration that he did not want to follow in his successful siblings' footsteps. Frank referred to them as "the perfects."

In tracing their family genealogy with the Wilsons, the social worker learned that Andrea's maternal grandparents had immigrated from Ireland. She grew up in a cohesive Roman Catholic family of seven and described herself and her siblings as "good kids who were happy to stay home and stay out of trouble." She could not recall being rebellious and seemed to have an idealized view of her parents as unselfishly hard-working and consistently loving—"I don't remember them ever raising their voices at us—they didn't need to." Andrea was a virgin when she married Michael, her high school sweetheart and the only man she had ever dated. Both her parents were deceased; she became tearful talking about her mother's death a year before: "I can't believe she's gone. We talked on the phone every day at least once. It's left a big hole in my heart."

Michael's parents were of Norwegian descent. He described them as stern, quiet people who rarely expressed their feelings. He had one sibling, a sister 10 years his senior, who lived in another state and with whom he rarely communicated. Despite advanced age and frailty, his parents continued to live in their own home near the Wilsons. They kept to themselves and, although Michael looked in on them monthly, there was little interaction otherwise. Given Andrea's experience of closeness with her own family, she found Michael's distance puzzling and referred to his parents as "strange."

There was a family tragedy in Michael's family's past—his paternal grandfather, a farmer, had committed suicide when Michael was 5 years old. He was told that his grandfather had a stroke and did not learn "the secret" until his sister told him when he was 15. Apparently the grandfather was frequently "down in the dumps," but no one knew his depression was so serious. Hearing this, Frank perked up and exclaimed, "You never told me that!" Michael also reported that his father's younger brother was being treated for depression and that his father was often moody as well. Andrea interjected here, "You're not always that perky yourself!"

Michael, always a shy, quiet youngster, was drawn in high school to Andrea's bubbly, outgoing personality: "I guess we were a good match." Because Andrea objected to marrying outside her faith, Michael agreed to convert to Catholicism. Asked how he felt about this, Michael shrugged and replied, "Oh, it was all right. I didn't think about it much. I didn't really agree with everything about the church—still don't—but it seemed to make her happy." Hearing this, Andrea raised her eyebrows in surprise.

For the fourth interview, the social worker was surprised to find Michael and Andrea in the waiting room alone, sans Frank. Asked where he was, they said he refused to come: "He says we're the ones with the problem! Can you believe it?" Thinking to herself that Frank might be right and that his acting out was probably a misdirected but age-appropriate effort to separate from his parents, the social worker said, "I imagine it's been hard for Frank to be here. He's at an age when he's trying to break away, and his refusal to come may be part of that effort. This is not at all unusual with the families I see. Even though he doesn't want to keep coming, I think that the three of us can keep working on the problem without him."

At first, the Wilsons took their customary chairs, leaving Frank's now empty chair in between them. Noticing that Andrea was looking anxiously at the chair, the social worker commented, "It must feel strange to be here without Frank." Andrea nodded, and Michael shifted uncomfortably in his seat. The worker then said, "I'd like to rearrange things a bit." She got up and removed Frank's chair from between the couple and asked them to move their chairs around so that they were almost facing each other. Hesitating a moment, they did so, looking somewhat stiff, almost formal. Asked how this new arrangement felt, Andrea said, "It feels funny. I even have some butterflies!" Michael looking awkward, said, "Yeah—it's odd without Frank."

For the first several couple sessions, the Wilsons kept their focus on their distress about Frank's shenanigans. Andrea declared, "Sometimes I think he's just plain mean. He does this to hurt us on purpose. I don't know where he got this mean streak. I'm about to give up on him and let him ruin his own life." The worker said, "I know Frank is giving you a really hard time, but I'm not sure why you're feeling so pessimistic. He's clearly testing the limits of your patience, but he seems to be basically a good kid." Andrea replied, "Well, *you* lie awake till 2:00 in the morning waiting for him to come home safe after you've told him his curfew is midnight!" The worker continued, "I imagine that must be very difficult. It sounds like it's hard for you not knowing where he is. What's it like?" Andrea sighed before saying, "I try to read, but basically I'm waiting for the phone to ring with the police on the other end. And Michael here is snoring along as usual." The worker said, "So you feel pretty alone with your fears." Andrea nodded and appeared tearful. This interaction marked a "heightened affective moment" (Beebe & Lachmann, 2002) that spoke to both Wilsons' feelings and strengthened the therapeutic alliance.

Turing to Michael, the worker then said, "I guess I'm hearing you don't have the same worries Andrea has." Shaking his head slowly, Michael said, "No—I sowed a few wild oats myself before I met Andrea. My parents didn't seem to care much if I stayed out, and I never got into trouble." The worker replied, "I wonder if you appreciate just how upset Andrea gets over Frank's behavior." Michael, shrugging, said, "I guess she gets pretty wired about it. I don't know how to help her calm down." The worker then asked Andrea what Michael could say or do that might help her feel more comfortable when she worried about Frank. Andrea said, "Well, it would help sometimes if he just said something like you did a minute ago, 'I know it's hard for you. I'm sorry you're so upset.'" The worker asked Michael if he could say that to Andrea now, in the session, and, haltingly, but sustaining eye contact with Andrea, he did so.

Over the next several sessions, the social worker began to encourage the Wilsons to communicate their feelings and thoughts to each other while she titrated her role as intermediary. As this process evolved, it became clear to the worker that there had always been considerable emotional distance between the two. At times they seemed like awkward teenagers on a blind date. The worker asked at one point, "How does it feel to be doing this without a coach?" Andrea replied, "I always thought we communicated really well. But when I think about it now, it was always around something going on with the kids." The worker said, "Your children began arriving right away, and often when that happens, couples focus so much on them that they have little time to work on their own relationship. With Frank getting ready to leave the nest, you have time to do some of that work now."

At this point the social worker introduced some communication and experiential exercises. As a homework assignment, the Wilsons were instructed to set aside a half hour three times during the next week to discuss each partner's perception of the positive and negative aspects of their marriage. Each partner was to have 10 minutes to speak without interruption from the other. This assignment was intended to increase in each partner awareness of the other's needs and feelings while also helping both think about and articulate their own. They were also asked to record their reflections on these interchanges in a journal.

Reporting that their homework felt very uncomfortable at first, by the end of the week the Wilsons were adapting well to it. Both noticed that they had little trouble listing the positives about each other but struggled with negative feelings. Continuing this assignment into a second week, they began to venture some complaints. In a subsequent session at the agency, Andrea confronted her husband: "You made me furious Saturday. Frank was lying around watching TV when he was supposed to be mowing the grass. I asked you to speak to him and, instead, you went out and cut the grass yourself!" The social worker asked Michael how it felt to hear this. He shrugged and said, with a sense of resignation, "It's just too much trouble to get him to do anything. It's easier to do it myself." Turning to Andrea, he continued, "You make me feel like you always know the right way to deal with him. I figure I'll just leave it to you."

The social worker congratulated the Wilsons for their courage in expressing their disappointment and anger at each other. She then instructed them in the use of "I" statements: "Rather than starting 'You made me furious' or 'You make me feel like such and such,' try beginning with 'I.' In these examples, it might sound like, 'I feel furious when you don't take a stand with Frank,' or 'I feel like you're the expert with Frank.'" This technique was intended to help the Wilsons "own" or take responsibility for, their own feelings rather than ascribing causation to the other.

Over several weeks, the Wilsons became more comfortable discussing a wider range of affects. Their now solid therapeutic alliance with the worker helped them talk more directly with each other while not turning to her as frequently. Over many sessions, longstanding disappointments emerged. Andrea had always found what she called Michael's passivity irritating. This trait expressed itself not just with the children but socially as well. His down moods and shyness had had a dampening effect on their social life. She felt embarrassed by his obvious discomfort with others outside the family, and they rarely went out. A gregarious person, Andrea found this difficult but had "accepted" it as something Michael could not change.

In exploring this behavior, it became clearer to the social worker that Michael suffered from chronic dysthymia interspersed with more pronounced bouts of depression. Considering his family history of depression, she suspected that there was likely a genetic component and referred him to the agency's consulting psychopharmacologist. The psychopharmacologist prescribed one of the SSRIs (selective serotonin reuptake inhibitors), and after about a month the worker noticed that Michael's facial features seemed more animated and that he had become more vocal in sessions. In addition to reporting that he was feeling "better than I have in years," he began expressing more anger toward Andrea. He reported longstanding anger about her insistence that they not practice birth control, a condition that had inhibited their sexual life considerably. With the arrival of each child he worried about the strain on the family finances. Although he had never told her, while Andrea was ec-static when she learned about her pregnancy with Frank, he at first be-came angry about it and, feeling guilty, later became quite depressed. He resented that only the children seemed to make her happy and that she had little affection left over for him.

Although Andrea became angry and defensive at first, with the social worker's help she was able to hear Michael out. Both partners gained in-creasing tolerance for ambivalence in their relationship. Meanwhile, the worker became more convinced that Frank's acting out had resulted, in part, from being the recipient of projected angry impulses that his parents could not express directly to each other. As they became more skilled at, and comfortable with, expressing their affects, Frank's acting out began to subside. The worker interpreted to the couple that, disappointed in aspects of their marriage, they may have gained a sense of well-being from their children's accomplishments. In that sense, the children were a buffer be-tween them that postponed their having to experience negative feelings and deal with each other more directly. At this point, the social worker recalled for the Wilsons that this "buffering" function had found a literal expression in the first appointment, when they had placed Frank between them.

To counter this role in the family structure, Frank had to find more forceful ways to separate. The frightening prospect of his separating and leaving the Wilsons "alone" led them to provoke Frank further by impos-ing increased restrictions and treating him, as he put it in an early family session, "like a baby." The prospect of "losing" Frank was particularly dif-ficult for Andrea, who was managing unresolved grief over her mother's death. Meanwhile, Frank's rebellious anger, while consciously distressing to them, also served the purpose of keeping both partners' unexpressed anger out of awareness.

Such systems-oriented formulations appeared to help the Wilsons be less critical of Frank and to listen to his thoughts and aspirations without imposing their own agenda for him. Unlike his idealized "perfect" sib-lings, he continued to get into minor scrapes from time to time, but An-drea and Michael's increased understanding of the family dynamics and their growing reliance on each other for affective expression helped them be more tolerant and less provocative.

PSYCHONEUROBIOLOGICAL SUBSTRATE
OF A FAMILY THERAPY CASE

The techniques employed by the social worker with the Wilsons are typical of family systems interventions. At the beginning, she concentrated on joining the family system, paid attention to the way the family structured itself in her office, noted body language, and, using the genogram, attended to intergenerational issues that might be influencing the family. Clinicians using a systems approach look at the whole family as the "client" and recognize that, during helping efforts, they also become part of the family system and, from that position, can influence its relational dynamics. Adding a neurobiological perspective to traditional family systems concepts helps clinicians appreciate the complex biopsychosocial nature of this influence.

As documented in previous chapters, the human brain is a social brain. From birth onward, the neural networks of the brain develop and become integrated in the context of affective interactions with others. Early, neurally encoded working models of attachment influence the nature of, and become revised in, the intimate arena of family life. Family systems clinicians believe that working in the affectively intense "heat" of here-and-how family conflict offers unique opportunities for catalyzing change.

The social worker's first objective for the Wilsons was to construct a holding environment wherein the family could feel safe in the clinical encounter. As Winnicott (1965d) suggested, such an environment must be optimally gratifying and optimally frustrating if development is to proceed. By noting but not commenting on the Wilsons' seating arrangement in the first few interviews, the worker permitted them to structure the clinical system in the way that felt most familiar. She listened quietly and attentively while Frank's parents ventilated their feelings about his behavior. She did not push Frank to talk before he seemed ready, thus gratifying his need for differentiation from his parents and her. In contrast, she instituted some frustration by imposing communication rules intended to help the family begin to postpone affective expression and modulate its intensity.

The worker's request that family members feed back what they heard each other saying was also intended to help them reflect on what they heard, toward the goal of enhancing their capacity for mentalization (Fonagy et al., 2002). A neuroscientist considering this intervention might conclude that, by interrupting the Wilsons' typical pattern of jumping in to make value judgments about what they heard, the worker was trying to enhance their cognitive control over automatic affective reactions, thus enhancing neural network integration. Later, teaching the Wilsons the technique of using "I" statements could also be seen as fostering such integration.

The genogram could be viewed as serving a similar purpose. Helping the family take some distance from the immediacy of their anxiety by charting their intergenerational heritage drew on their cognitive capacities. This exercise also served a psychoeducational purpose as the worker pointed out interesting family patterns and mused about their impact on the Wilsons' current family life. Learning about the history of depression in Michael's family and about Andrea's continuing grief over her mother's death helped the worker appreciate biological and stress-related components of family issues. Aware of the genetically determined biological components of depression, for example, she instituted a medication evaluation that eventuated in Michael getting relief from years of dysthymia.

The homework assignments could also be conceptualized as efforts to enhance neural network integration and affect tolerance. From this perspective, the structured assignments created affectively "safe emergencies" (Cozolino, 2002), intended to activate a moderate degree of anxiety in both Wilsons but in a situation that felt bounded and safe. As noted earlier, high levels of affect block thinking, whereas moderate levels foster the integration of cognition and affect. Setting a time limit for sharing thoughts and feelings helped keep their anxiety at moderate levels. Having them write in a journal about their responses to the assignment further called on cognitive processing capacities to help modulate the intensity of affect-laden experiences. Cozolino concluded that such traditional family systems techniques "increase cortical involvement with previously reflexive and regressive emotions and behaviors. [Furthermore,] . . . psychological, interpersonal, and neural integration are different manifestations of the same process" (2002, p. 59).

CONCLUSION

Each of these case studies exemplifies solid, relationally based clinical social work practice. By weaving knowledge from neurobiology into the assessment and intervention processes described, we have attempted to convey ways in which this knowledge can broaden and deepen the biopsychosocial approach of social work. The "heightened affective moments" depicted in each example resonate with Perlman's assertion, quoted in Chapter 1 and again here, that "relationship leaps from one person to the other at the moment when emotion moves between them" (1957, p. 65). Findings from neurobiology provide evidence that this "leap" occurs at the neurological level. Each of the interventions described is based on the principle of neural plasticity. This principle conveys optimism that even longstanding, neurally encoded habits of brain and mind can be positively altered in attuned clinical relationships.

Chapter 10

NEW DIRECTIONS FOR SOCIAL WORK EDUCATION

THE PRIMARY PURPOSE of this chapter is to examine the ways in which recent research on the social context of brain development in early life can be integrated into several curricular areas of social work education. In addition, we consider ways in which this body of work can be utilized by students to inform new research questions in social work as well as to prepare them to advocate for social policies focused on the well-being of children and families. Moreover, because social workers so often work with other allied disciplines, such as education and medicine, we consider how future generations of social workers may be able to utilize this research to inform collaborations focused on supporting the strengths of children and families.

A central focus in social work education is the delivery of content that acquaints students with a biopsychosocial perspective on understanding and assisting people they encounter in the various setting in which they will practice. Recent models of risk and resiliency highlight the ways in which biological, psychological, and social factors combine to shape the trajectories of human development (Fraser, 1997; Shonkoff & Phillips,

2000). Yet the biological dimension of this tripartite perspective is frequently underdeveloped in social work education. This absence has become particularly noticeable as research in developmental biology and the cognitive neurosciences has continued to shed light on the multifaceted nature of development in both children and adults (Cicchetti & Cohen, 1995). As we have reviewed throughout this volume, of particular relevance to social work education and practice are those studies that illuminate the processes of brain development in early life (Nelson & Bloom, 1997; Shonkoff & Phillips, 2000) and the ways in which various aspects of brain development are critical components of social and emotional well-being (Schore, 1997a). In addition, studies in developmental neurobiology and the cognitive neurosciences have made important contributions to our understanding of *plasticity*, or the capacity for regeneration, recovery, and change across the lifespan (Shonkoff & Phillips, 2000).

Neurobiological development is both hierarchical and complex, shaped by the environment *and* a full complement of intrinsic and health-related factors. Although the study of brain development in early life certainly blurs the boundaries between "nature" and "nurture," this research itself is still in its infancy. Researchers and clinicians are now beginning to examine empircally the ways in which early life experience affects brain development and, in turn, how the neurobiological substrate of early experience is carried forward over time in many aspects of human behavior and development. In this volume, we have focused primarily on the influence of early relational experience in shaping the neurobiological substrate of, and hence capacity for, affect regulation. This area was chosen because the ability to regulate affect is a key factor in maintaining coping, adaptation, and mental health.

The capacity for affect regulation, an important part of emotional development in early life, emerges in the context of important caregiving relationships and becomes hard-wired into the neuronal structure of the developing brain (Shapiro & Applegate, 2000). Early relational experience, or nurturance, has been identified as a primary factor that operates in conjunction with variables such as adequate nutrition and freedom from abuse and neglect to promote healthy brain development. In order todelineate the

ways in which this complex body of research may be integrated into social work education, it is necessary to consider how these studies reflect
the biopsychosocial perspective and, in particular, how the person-in-
environment, or ecological, perspective typically associated with social
work education is useful in considering the application of this research to
various areas and levels of social work practice, research, and policy.

The urgency and timeliness of incorporating the above aspects of neuroscience into social work education are underscored by recent findings
that the sequelae of affectively dysregulated caregiving experiences can
be severe and long-lasting (Beebe & Lachman, 1988; Goldstein & Goldstein, 1996; Hughes, Catania, Derevensky, & Dongier, 1997; Perry, 1995)
and may be transmitted across generations (Crandall et al., 1997). Many
populations of parents and children with whom social workers come into
contact are at risk for dyresgulated interaction. For example, as described
in Chapter 7, children of depressed parents, children whose parents are
substance abusing, or children who have experienced traumatic early beginnings (e.g., in the child welfare system) do not have access to the kind
of sensitive, attuned, and empathic caregiving that is associated with developmental competence in a range of spheres. Further, we began the mil-
lennium facing changes in welfare reform that may threaten the integrity
of early caregiving environments for infants and children, as more primary caregivers enter the workforce without access to affordable quality
child care (Galinsky, 1998).

The remainder of this chapter is divided into three sections. First, we
present an overview of several concepts and methods germane to the study
of neurobiology and the cognitive neurosciences. The concepts chosen
for review have particularly salient implications for enhancing the biological dimension of the tripartite biopsychosocial perspective more typical of social work education and practice. Second, we briefly review the
manner in which early brain development is shaped by relational experience and associated with the capacity for affect regulation, itself a core element of mental health and the capacity for adaptation. Third, we discuss
specific ways in which insights from new research in developmental neurobiology can be used to enhance the core content areas of social work
education.

IDEAS AND METHODS FROM BRAIN RESEARCH

Many ideas and methods derived from recent multidisciplinary study of brain development, structure, organization, and function have applied utility for social work education and practice. Although beyond the scope of this chapter to provide a detailed review, we have chosen several concepts most salient to illuminating processes of development and risk and resiliency in infancy and early childhood.

Optimal Development

There has been rapid progress in understanding how the brain develops and, in particular, the extremely rapid changes in brain development that occur both prenatally and in the early years of life (Shonkoff & Phillips, 2000). Much of this work has focused on the identification of a range of biopsychosocial variables that influence aspects of brain development. This research has particular relevance to social work education, because many at-risk populations with whom social workers come into contact share characteristics identified as posing risks to healthy brain development. Among the most noted of these characteristics are exposure to environmental toxins, poor maternal nutrition, maternal stress, family violence, poverty, and exposure to other teratogens such as alcohol and drugs. These variables can operate directly on the developing brain but may also provide indirect influence via their impact on other important factors, such as the quality of early caregiving given to the developing child. As we have discussed, the quality of early caregiving has emerged as an important influence on postnatal brain development (Schore, 1994, 1997a; Perry, 1995).

From the perspective of social work education, this research is important because it contributes to students' understanding of the ways in which developmental outcomes considered to be "biological" in nature (i.e., based in brain development) may be shaped by various aspects of the environment. This blurring of the traditional boundary between "nature" and "nurture" is important for social work students to consider, as they traverse between person and environment in the conceptualization of both preventive and tertiary interventions.

Neural Plasticity

The concept of neural plasticity provides a balanced view of the importance of early experience in relation to a belief in the capacity for change. Social work students must be encouraged to form views of human behavior that are based on (1) a belief in the role of early experience, and (2) a belief in the capacity for change and recovery via altered situational characteristics or therapeutic intervention. Thus it is important, for many reasons, for students to understand the concept of neural plasticity, which refers to the extent to which the developing brain is influenced by a range of environmental factors (Nelson & Bloom, 1997); more specifically, the way in which neural connections in the brain may reorganize following exposure to either positive or negative experience, First, research on neural plasticity is an important antidote to the common view of the brain as being rigidly determined by genetic history, set in its developmental trajectory and unresponsive to environmental influences. From the perspective of social work education, the concept of neural plasticity supports the idea of change via altered situational characteristics and therapeutic intervention. And yet, as is pointed out by Shonkoff and Phillips (2000), the concept of neural plasticity is a "double-edged sword" because, by highlighting the ways in which the developing brain is open to environmental influence, our attention is also drawn to the great potential vulnerability of children in high-risk environments. Thus, the construct of neural plasticity not only informs our understanding of risk and protective processes in infancy and childhood but also highlights the importance of early assessment and intervention and of programs that support the well-being of young children and their families.

The Centrality of Early Childhood

As described in Chapter 1, the brain develops rapidly during the sensitive period of the first 3 years of life. Although evidence indicates that the brain retains a degree of plasticity throughout life, early childhood experience is particularly salient because the organization and structure of the brain are still in their crucial formative stages. It is during these formative stages that the connective "wiring" of the social brain occurs.

Types of Early Experience and the Nature of Neuronal Connections

As described in Chapter 1, the manner in which synaptic connections among neurons is fomed is both "experience-dependent" and "experience-expectant" (Greenough & Black, 1992; Nelson & Bloom, 1997). An understanding of these concepts enables students to appreciate the significance of early relational input for optimal brain development.

Advances in the Methods of Neuropsychology and Neuroimaging

Increasingly sophisticated empirical methods in neuropsychology and neuroimaging have made it possible to study the anatomical structure and function of the brain with increasing specificity (Nelson & Bloom, 1997). We reviewed these methods in some detail in Chapter 1. Although students do not need to know the technical specificities of these methods, it is helpful to acquaint them with the ways in which conclusions about brain structure and functioning are determined. These methodologies have helped to delineate the neurological bases, or substrates, of normative processes such as learning and problem solving as well as clinical entities such as Alzheimer's disease (Selkoe, 1998), and the impact of trauma on brain development (Post et al., 1997), and the ways in which unmediated experiences of childhood physical or sexual abuse may be reflected in brain organization and structure (Stein, Hanna, Koverola, & Torchia, 1997).

DEVELOPMENTAL THEORY, NEUROBIOLOGY, AND SOCIAL WORK EDUCATION AND PRACTICE

As described throughout this volume, early relational experience becomes a determinant of the neurobiological substrates of affect regulation, relational capacity, and mental health. In addition, the capacity for affect regulation is central to many of the components that comprise "school readiness," such as attention, cognition, and learning (Noshpitz & King, 1991). Moreover, as illustrated in the case studies of Chapter 9, there is growing evidence that affect regulation styles are transmitted across generations via their manifestation in the caregiving environment (Crandall et al., 1997; Roumell, Wille, Abramson, & Delaney, 1997). For example, a depressed mother is likely to have a reduced repertoire of affects to "teach" to her infant, and at the same time, is likely to be less "emotionally available" (Emde, 1985), creating an environment in which infant cues may be misread or ignored, or in which the caregiver herself is either over- or understimulating in her behavior toward the infant, resulting in affective dysregulation, or dyssynchrony, between infant and caregiver (Stern, 1985).

Many populations of parents and infants with whom social work students will come into contact are at risk, due to a complex array of biological and psychosocial factors, for dysregulation in the parent–infant relationship and, relatedly, for disturbances in the child's capacity to regulate strong feelings. As is suggested by process models of parenting (Belsky, 1984), this dysregulation can stem from the interaction of parental, child, and contextual variables. In addition to the psychological, neurological, and physical well-being of the parent and the health status, temperament, and neurological idiosyncrasies of the child, a myriad of contextual factors, such as the degree of environmental stress or support, may combine to influence a family's style of regulating intense affect within a relational context. Variables such as parental psychopathology, young maternal age, family violence, substance abuse, childhood illness, and chronic poverty may create transactional environments that pose challenges to the capacity of the parent–infant dyad to establish affectively regulated interaction patterns. To consider this wide range of variables, social work students must develop a multisystemic conceptual framework. This framework, with the inclusion of neurobiological variables, can inform courses in both theory and practice.

IMPLICATIONS FOR SOCIAL WORK EDUCATION

Research on brain development in early life, such as that presented here, requires a new conceptual integration of the biological and psychosocial processes that shape, and result from, the earliest interactions between the developing infant and his or her caregiving environment. Key to this inquiry is a deepened comprehension of the ways in which people learn to regulate their strongest feelings and, in turn, teach what they have learned to those infants and children in their care. Knowledge derived from this research is relevant to curriculum development in several core areas of social work education, including the human behavior and the social environment sequence, courses in foundation and advanced direct practice, and child- and family-focused electives. In the following section, we discuss the ways in which this content supports the training of practitioners at multiple systems levels and underscores the importance and meaning of the helping relationship.

Human Behavior and The Social Environment

The Council on Social Work Education (CSWE) Curriculum Policy Statement for Master's Programs mandates that human behavior and social environment (HBSE) courses provide content about human biological, psychological, and social development, including theories and knowledge about the various social systems in which people live. A primary goal of many HBSE courses is to consider various conceptualizations of human development and behavior and the ways in which theory can be applied to social work practice in a variety of settings. As research on the biological substrate of human behavior continues to become more nuanced, the traditional boundaries between "nature" and "nurture" continue to blur, requiring an increased capacity to examine the ways in which biological, psychological, and social factors transact to create unique contexts for the developing individual.

Social work students need conceptual frameworks that support the integration of findings from the biological sciences into models of risk and resiliency, and of human behavior and development. Many frameworks are multisystemic in nature and support multidimensional assessments and intervention planning. In addition, the person-in-environment and ecological perspectives support students' ability to consider the nature of the transactions between individuals and their surrounding environments on multiple levels. In order to integrate research described in this volume, students must be capable of integrating a range of individual, familial, and societal determinants of development *and* of understanding the ways in which such factors form complex matrices that particularize the developmental context of each child and family. Toward this end, frameworks such as Fraser's (1997) multisystemic model of risk and resilience and Bronfenbrenner's (1979) model of the social ecology of human development are particularly useful.

Fraser describes an ecological and multisystemic perspective that identifies a matrix of factors that influence processes of risk and resiliency in development. These factors include (1) broad environmental conditions, (2) family, school, and neighborhood conditions, and (3) individual psychosocial and biological characteristics (Fraser, 1997, p. 20). Recent research in the cognitive neurosciences suggests that brain development is related to factors in each of these clusters and, more specifically, that aspects of these clusters interact to shape the neurobiological substrate of developmental well-being. In this regard, aspects of Bronfenbrenner's (1979) schema for conceptualizing the ecology of human development are also relevant. Namely, Bronfenbrenner defined multiple contexts of human development that were "conceived as a set of nested structures, each inside the next, like a set of Russian dolls" (p. 3). Bronfenbrenner's model describes the ways in which variables at multiple environmental levels transact to create particularized contexts for human behavior and development. In Bronfenbrenner's model, four "levels" of social ecology are described: microystem, mesosystem, exosystem, and macrosystem.

At the innermost level, the *microsystem*, the focus of inquiry is on the pattern of activities, roles, and relationships experienced directly by the developing person. As amply documented above, the key aspect of the microsystemic environment that emerges as important in understanding the neurobiology of affect regulation is the pattern of relational transactions between the infant and his or her immediate caregivers, typically the parents. Here the focus is on the level of affective attunement between caregivers and infant—the degree to which caregivers can accurately "read" and appropriately respond to the baby's first socioemotional expressions. Thus, any parental, child, or contextual factors that support or impede the achievement of affective attunement between parent and infant are relevant to this discussion. In addition to learning about the psychology of bonding and attachment, students introduced to findings from neuroscience come to appreciate the neurobiological substrate and consequences of these relational phenomena. As an example, child abuse represents a profound dysregulation of affect in the context of the infant–caregiver relationship. One example of affect dysregulation appears when the caregiver, unable to control his or her own reaction to a baby's persistent crying, strikes out in physical abuse, thus escalating the baby's distress in ways that may further dysregulate the caregiver and the caregiver–infant interaction. The research reviewed here suggests that, if persistent and unmediated, such patterns of dysregulated interaction may become neurologically imprinted in ways that influence the developing child's ability to utilize the primary caregiver as a "secure base" (Bowlby, 1988) from which to explore the human and object world.

Similarly, parents' efforts to modulate affective expression may result in understimulation of babies, as might be the case when a parent neglects a child for fear of being unable to modulate emotional arousal in relationship to the dependence of a developing infant. In either case, an unmediated pattern of dysregulated interaction may color subsequent interactions between the baby and others with anxiety and a mistrustful approach to relationships. Curriculum development in this area might focus not only on the integration of this research, but on the introduction of observational assessment methods that support the social worker's ability to assess the caregiver–infant relationship in a context-responsive manner, and that support the development of early intervention methods.

At the next ecological level, the *mesosystem*, attention is focused on the transactions among two or more elements in the developing baby's environment. An important example here exists in the direct and indirect ways in which interactions between the baby's parents, or between any primary caregiver and significant others, may influence the developing child. We know from cognitive–behavioral theory and research that modeling plays a crucial role in shaping children's interactional style and manner of managing intense feelings. If routinely exposed to an environment wherein caregivers' affective interactions are characterized by dysregulation (e.g., outbursts of anger, physical violence, or the blunted affective repertoire of chronic depression), babies are likely to observe, take in, and, as these findings would suggest, "encode" neurologically what they experience. For students studying internalization and identification, the idea that these psychological processes have neurological correlates in brain development renders them less abstract and mysterious. Students can also be encouraged to look at transactional environments beyond the immediate family setting, such as can be found in out-of-home child care. Child-care centers are often characterized by large group sizes, low ratios of caregivers to children, rapid turnover of staff, low pay, and little access to ongoing training (Phillips, Howes, & Whikbook, 2002). These characteristics pose great challenges to child-care providers and infants alike. For the child care staff, it is a challenge to manage their own affects and relationally very demanding to come to "know" individual infants well enough to empathically recognize and respond to the babies' emotional states and needs—which are, of course, communicated nonverbally.

The *exosystem* is comprised of those elements or settings that may not involve the developing baby as an active participant but which may ultimately influence his or her development both directly and indirectly. Such factors as parents' work status, neighborhood conditions, and the nature of the family's social support system take on significance here. For example, if work environments offer little flexibility or consistency, parents may face great challenges in managing their own stress levels and in keeping attuned to individual infant characteristics, such as temperament, and the overall emotional lives of their infants. Moreover, many children with whom social workers come into contact grow up in chaotic environments where unemployment, poverty, and societal violence prevail. Such conditions impact caregivers' capacity to attend mindfully to their children's emotional needs, including their need for recognition of, and responsive attunement to, their varying feeling states. Such children may become the targets of displaced frustration and anger or may be left alone—that is, over- or understimulated in ways that compromise their capacity to regulate affects adaptively.

The outermost level of the nested arrangement of concentrically depicted systemic structures in Bronfenbrenner's schema is the *macrosystem*, or the larger patterns produced by consistencies in the previously described lower-order systems and which find expression in culturally grounded belief systems and ideologies. Here students can examine the ideological and philosophical underpinnings of social policies directed to children's well-being and their impact on child development generally and neurobiological development specifically. For example, much as been written about the importance of early parent–child interaction in relationship to cognitive mastery and "school readiness" from birth to 5 years of age. Less has been written about the affective experience of the child's early life and the ways in which caregiver–child interaction patterns can support cognitive capacity by helping the child to learn to regulate emotional arousal. In addition, interesting questions for discussion can be generated by the likely impact on children's brain development of this culture's emphasis on the timely achievement of cognitive and socioemotional milestones and the distress and frustration communicated by parents whose children may not meet the desired standards "on time." Other relevant questions emerge in discussion of the philosophical assumptions behind current foster-care practices, especially those leading to multiple placements and inconsistency among caregiving environments.

In order to fully appreciate the complex, transacting, and often apparently chaotic nature of these systemic elements, students can be introduced to the theory of nonlinear dynamics, or complexity theory, detailed in Chapter 4. An excellent overview of this theory is provided in Hudson's (2000) article, titled "At the Edge of Chaos: A New Paradigm for Social Work?" in the *Journal of Social Work Education*.

Foundation and Advanced Practice Courses

Students in both foundation and advanced practice courses are well served by efforts that encourage an integration of person-in-environment perspectives with a biopsychosocial view of human development. From a social work perspective, it is possible for students to incorporate emerging research in the cognitive neurosciences into their understanding of the social ecology of human development and the ways in which multiple variables interact to shape important developmental contexts. Bronfenbrenner's (1979) comprehensive model for examining the ecology of the person-in-environment can also guide the incorporation of this content into courses in direct social work practice.

At the micropractice level, the research reviewed here offers new ways to understand the processes by which the helping relationship potentiates changes and healing. Social workers have long recognized the importance of the helping relationship in successful intervention outcomes. It is within the context of a helping relationship that is supportive and infused with an empathic understanding of the client's mental state that processes of change and healing are potentiated. This kind of "clinical caring" (Imre, 1982) is central to the helping process.

As noted, although we know that early brain development persists in neuronal structure, research suggests that a degree of plasticity remains throughout the lifespan. There is growing evidence that attuned clinical intervention can take advantage of this plasticity by altering brain structure and chemistry in beneficial ways (Gabbard, 1992). Spezzano (1993), for example, suggested that attuned clinicians facilitate right-brain development by attending to the methods by which clients have regulated their affective states and modeling new ways of affective response. The crisis-ridden client, for example, can internalize less dysregulated ways of managing intense feeling states through empathic resonance with, and mirroring by, a clinician presenting a calm, focused, and modulated demeanor. In addition, introducing students to Cozolino's (2002) clinical strategies for promoting neural network integration can enhance their understanding of how effective helping relationships affect the brain. Learning that neural network integration enhances adaptive affect regulation, students gain clinical tools that help them promote clients' resilience and competencies to preserve nonchaotic interpersonal environments, even when external circumstances are chaotic.

At the mesosystemic level, workers who assess and intervene with families can employ aspects of family theory and practice that address the transmission of patterns of affect regulation across generations. An appreciation of the extent to which such patterns become part of a family's neurobiological heritage can help students understand their persistence and develop relationship-based strategies for promoting more adaptive affect regulation. A practice focus on the exosystem can prepare students to become careful observers of affect regulation patterns in such field placement settings as schools, child welfare agencies, adoption agencies, and pediatric medical facilities. Systemic assessments based on such observation can help them use their skills to promote agency policies and programs that are sensitive to the ways in which expressions of intense feelings are addressed. Finally, the macrosystemic arena of social ideology and policy provides the context for helping students attend to prevention through such initiatives as parent education programs, psychoeducational training for child-care workers, and social action and advocacy for children and families at risk for affect dysregulation and its detrimental neurobiological sequelae. Electives in both micro- and macro-practice can broader and deepen students' awareness of the extent to which the neurobiology of dysregulated affect plays a part in such issues as mental illness, posttraumatic stress, substance abuse, and in both domestic and societal violence.

Incorporating Research on Brain Development in Early Life

As we have discussed elsewhere, research on brain development in early life is an interdisciplinary field that requires the capacity to integrate findings from many areas of study. From the perspective of social work education, the burgeoning fields of developmental neurobiology and cognitive neuroscience require social work students to become familiar enough with the language and concepts of these fields to be able to *read* about new research and *understand* the implications of this research for the conceptualization of risk and resiliency and for social work practice and policy. This task does not require each social work student or practitioner to become "expert" in the field of neuroscience, because excellent resources exist that describe, in clear language, the core elements of this field of work and the import of current research for the study of human behavior.

Research from neurobiology and the cognitive neuroscience raises many important questions for social workers and other professionals who work to support optimal development and functioning in children and families. First, the study of early brain development shines a spotlight on the role of early experience in developmental well-being. For clinicians this research underscores the importance of early assessment and intervention. In the realm of policy, this research points to the importance of programs and policies that support families in their efforts to provide stability, freedom from abuse and neglect, adequate nutrition, housing, and medical care, and both the time and psychological energy for engaging in stable and empathically attuned caregiving.

Second, research on brain development in early life encourages us to study anew the relationship between affect and cognitive capacity. In a culture focused on early achievement in the realm of "school readiness" and academic success, it is important that social work advocate for other allied disciplines to understand the relationship between affective well-being and both cognitive ability and academic performance.

Third, research on brain development in early life suggests that when early environments have been chaotic and disrupted, children may retain aspects of internal fragility even when a new environment that is "safer" and "more secure" is introduced. As we think about how to measure the "effectiveness" of interventions that focus on environmental changes (e.g., child welfare), it is important to consider how we think about and measure the degree of internal fragility a child may have subsequent to difficult early beginnings. Certainly, the research on brain development in early life suggests that neurological pathways that are established in response to the pattern of early care experiences may persist over time.

Tools for The Classroom

One challenge faced by social work educators is the identification of tools that can be helpful in the integration of this material into the classroom setting. It is our belief that social work students can think about this material from a variety of perspectives. One approach is to think about which core elements from the vast knowledge base of neurobiology are most relevant to social work education. Are there resources available that translate some of this knowledge base into language that is "user-friendly" for students and professionals who are not familiar with the language of neuroscience?

There has been substantial growth in the kinds of resources made available to help address the need for knowledge in this area. Perhaps the best example of this kind of research is the recent and widely circulated report titled *From Neurons to Neighborhood: The Science of Early Childhood Development* (Shonkoff & Phillips, 2000). Published by the National Research Council and the Institute of Medicine, this volume contains a chapter on "The Developing Brain" that summarizes, in easily understood language, research on areas such as (1) the specifics of early brain development, (2) postnatal neurogenesis, (3) the neurochemistry of early brain development, (4) how the brain is affected by early experience, and (5) the effect of early biological insults on the developing brain. Other resources easily available include many Web-based publications. Perhaps the most accessible of these is the section called "brain wonders" on the website of the "Zero to Three" organization (www.zerotothree.org), a national organization focused on promoting healthy development in infants and toddlers via encouraging the support of families and communities.

Students who seek to integrate this research into their professional development and practice must also develop observational skills that enable them to look for and understand nonverbal signs of affect regulation and dysregulation. The field of developmental psychology and research has developed a range of standardized observational methods to help researchers recognize various nonverbal cues of the emotional world of infants and young children. Clinicians have also described the importance of nonverbal signals as insights into the emotional world of children as well as adolescents and adults who may not be able to rely on the use of language to describe their emotional experience. Questions such as the following help focus the clinician's "eye" and thinking on the child's internal capacity for the regulation of affect, without necessarily knowing the "details" of the child's narrative:

1. What are the nonverbal signals of various mood states?
2. What nonverbal "coping strategies" does the child use when experiencing negative affective states?
3. How does the child use relationships (e.g., the parent caregiver, the clinician) in coping with states of affective arousal?
4. Does the child seem to rely on others for coping in constructive ways, or is the child more likely to withdraw into him- or herself?
5. How does it feel, as a clinician, to work with a particular child? What is your subjective reaction to the child when you spend time with him or her?

Emerging research in developmental neurobiology and the cognitive neurosciences provides an important complement to existing psychosocial studies on indicators of social and emotional development in infancy and childhood. This body of work adds a biological component to our understanding of the centrality of early caregiving quality in models of risk and resiliency in infancy, early childhood, and beyond. One aspect of this work that has received particular attention is the genesis of the capacity for affect regulation, or the ability to modulate emotional arousal. As we have discussed, this area of work is of particular relevance to social work education and practice, because sequelae associated with dysregulated affective experience are core features of many indicators of psychopathology in both childhood and adulthood. This work provides an important example of how the biological dimension of the biopsychosocial perspective can enhance students' understanding of models of human behavior and can inform effective strategies of multidimensional assessment and practice.

REFERENCES

Ainsworth, M. D. S., Blehar, M. C., Waters, E., & Wall, S. (1978). *Patterns of attachment: A psychological study of the Strange Situation*. Hillsdale, NJ: Erlbaum.

American Psychiatric Association. (1994). *Diagnostic and statistical manual of mental disorders* (4th ed.). Washington, DC: Author.

Applegate, J. S. (1993). Winnicott and clinical social work: A facilitating partnership. *Child and Adolescent Social Work Journal, 10,* 3–19.

Applegate, J. S. (2004). Full circle: Returning psychoanalytic theory to social work education. *Psychoanalytic Social Work, 11,* 23–36.

Applegate, J. S., & Bonovitz, J. M. (1995). *The facilitating partnership: A Winnicottian approach for social workers and other helping professionals*. Northvale, NJ: Jason Aronson.

Aron, L. (1996). *A meeting of minds: Mutuality in psychoanalysis*. Hillsdale, NJ: Analytic Press.

Beckwith, L. (1990). Adaptive and maladaptive parenting: Implications for intervention. In S. Meisels & J. Shonkoff (Eds.), *Handbook of early childhood intervention* (pp. 53–77). Cambridge, MA: Cambridge University Press.

Beebe, B., & Lachman, F. (1988). The contributions of mother–infant mutual influence to the origins of the self and object relationships. *Psychoanalytic Psychology, 5,* 305–307.

Beebe, B., & Lachmann, F. M. (2002). *Infant research and adult treatment: Co-constructing interactions*. Hillsdale, NJ: Analytic Press.

Beebe, B., & Stern, D. (1977). Engagement–disengagement and early object experiences. In N. Freedman & S. Grand (Eds.), *Communicative structures and psychic structures* (pp. 35–55). New York: Plenum Press.

Begley, S. (2002, October 11). Survival of the busiest. *Wall Street Journal,* pp. B1, B4.

Belsky, J. (1984). The determinants of parenting: A process model. *Child Development, 55,* 83–96.

Benedek, T. (1959). Parenthood as a developmental phase: A contribution to libido theory. *Journal of the American Psychoanalytic Association, 7,* 389–417.

Benoit, D., & Parker, K. (1994). Stability and transmission of attachment across three generations. *Child Development, 65,* 1444–1457.

Berger, R. L., McBreen, J. T., & Rifkin, M. J. (1996). *Human behavior: A perspective for the helping professions* (4th ed.). White Plains, NY: Longman.

Biestek, F. P. (1957). *The casework relationship*. Chicago: Loyola University Press.

Black, J., Jones, T., Nelson, C., & Greenough, W. (1998). Neruonal plasticity and the developing brain. In Alessi, N., Coyle, J., Harrison, S., & Eth, S. (Eds.), *Handbook of child and adolescent psychiatry*, Vol. 6, (pp. 31–53). NY: John Wiley.

Blos, P. (1967). The second individuation process of adolescence. *The Psychoanalytic Study of the Child, 22*, 162–186.

Bowlby, J. (1969). *Attachment and loss: Vol. 1. Attachment*. New York: Basic Books.

Bowlby, J. (1980). *Attachment and loss: Vol. 3. Loss*. New York: Basic Books.

Bowlby, J. (1988). *A secure base: Parent–child attachment and healthy human development*. New York: Basic Books.

Bradley, S. J. (2000). *Affect regulation and the development of psychopathology*. New York: Guilford Press.

Brazelton, T. B. (1992, May). *Touch and the fetus*. Presented to Gouch Research Institute, Miami, FL.

Bremner, J., & Narayan, M. (1998). The effects of stress on memory and the hippocampus throughout the life cycle: Implications for childhood development and aging. *Development and Psychopathology, 10*, 871–888.

Brenner, C. (1974). On the nature and development of affects: A unified theory. *Psychoanalytic Quarterly, 43*, 532–566.

Brenner, C. (1979). Working alliance, therapeutic alliance and transference. *Journal of the American Psychoanalytic Association, 27*, 137–157.

Bromberg, P. M. (2003). Something wicked this way comes: Trauma, dissociation, and conflict: The space where psychoanalysis, cognitive science and neuroscience overlap. *Psychoanalytic Psychology, 20*, 558–574.

Bronfenbrenner, U. (1979). *The ecology of human development: Experiments by nature and design*. Cambridge, MA: Harvard University Press.

Brooks-Gunn, J. (1990). Adolescents as daughters and as mothers: A developmental perspective. In I. Sigel & G. Brody (Eds.), *Methods of family research* (Vol. 1, pp. 213–248). Hillsdale, NJ: Erlbaum.

Brooks-Gunn, J., & Furstsenberg, F. (1986). The children of adolescent mothers: Physical, academic and psychological outcomes. *Developmental Review, 6*, 224–251.

Campbell, S., Cohn, J., & Neyers, T. (1995). Depression in first-time mothers: Mother–infant interaction and depression chronicity. *Developmental Psychology, 31*, 349–357.

Carlson, M., & Earls, F. (1997). Psychological and neuroendocrinological sequelae of early social deprivation in institutionalized children in Romania. *Annals of the New York Academy of Science, 807*, 419–428.

Carter, L., & Larson, C. (1997). Drug-exposed infants. *Future of Children, 7*, 157–160.

Carter, S., Osofsky, J., Hann, D. (1992). Speaking for the baby: A therapeutic intervention for odolescent mothers and their infants. *Infant Mental Health Journal, 12*(4), 291–301.

Cassidy, J. (1994). Emotion regulation: Influences of attachment relationships. *Monograph of the Society for Research in Child Development, 59*, 228–249.

Cassidy, J., & Shaver, P. (Eds.). (1999). *Handbook of attachment: Theory, research, and clinical implications*. New York: Guilford Press.

Chase-Lansdale, P., Brooks-Gunn, J., & Paikoff, R. (1991). Research and programs for adolescent mothers: Missing links and future promises. *Family Relations, 40*, 396–402.

Chasnoff, I., Anson, A., Hatcher, R., Stenson, H., & Iaukea, K. (1998). Prenatal exposure to cocaine and other drugs: Outcome at four to six years. In J. Harvey & B. Kosofsky (Eds.), *Cocaine: Effects on the developing brain. Annals of the New York Academy of Sciences, 846,* 314–328.

Chess, S., & Thomas, A. (1991). Temperament and the concept of goodness of fit. In J. Strelau & A. Angleitner (Eds.), *Explorations in temperament: International perspectives on theory and measurement* (pp. 15–28). New York: Plenum Press.

Cicchetti, D., & Cohen, D. (1995). *Perspectives on developmental psychopathology: Vol. 1. Theory and methods* (pp. 3–20). New York: Wiley.

Cicchetti, D., Rogosch, & Toth, S. (1998). Maternal depressive disorder and contextual risk. *Development and Psychopathology, 10,* 283–300.

Clore, G. L., & Ortony, A. (2000). Cognition in emotion: Always, sometimes, or never? In R. D. Lane & L. Nadel (Eds.), *Cognitive neuroscience of emotion* (pp. 24–61). New York: Oxford University Press.

Cohn, J., & Tronick, J. (1989). Specificity of infant's responsiveness to mother's affective behavior. *Journal of the American Academy of Child Psychiatry, 28,* 242–248.

Cote, J., & Levine, C. (1988). A critical examination of the ego identity status paradigm. *Developmental Review, 8,* 147–184.

Cozolino, L. (2002). *The neuroscience of psychotherapy: Building and rebuilding the human brain.* New York: Norton.

Crandall, L., Fitzgerald, H., & Whipple, E. (1997). Dyadic synchrony in parent–child interactions: A link with maternal representation of attachment relationships. *Infant Mental Health Journal, 18,* 247–264.

Culp, R., Culp, A., Osofsky, J., & Osofsky, H. (1991). Adolescent and older mothers' interaction patterns with their six-month-old infants. *Journal of Adolescence, 14,* 195–200.

Dacey, J., & Travers, J. (2002). Adolescence. In *Human development across the lifespan* (5th ed., pp. 274–332). New York: McGraw-Hill.

Damasio, A. R. (1994). *Descartes error: Emotion, reason, and the human brain.* New York: Grosset/Putnam.

Damasio, A. R. (1999). *The feeling of what happens: Body and emotion in the making of consciousness.* New York: Harcourt Brace.

Darwin, C. (1965). *The expression of emotions in man and animals.* Chicago: University of Chicago Press. (Original work published 1872)

Davidson, R., Ekman, P., Saron, C., Senulis, R., & Friesen, W. (1990). Approach-withdrawal and cerebral assymetry: Emotional expression and brain physiology. *Journal of Personality and Social Psychology, 58,* 330–341.

Dawson, S., Frey, K., Panagiotides, H., Osterling, J., & Hessl, D. (1997). Infants of depressed mothers exhibit atypical frontal brain activity: A replication and extension of previous findings. *Journal of Child Psychology and Psychiatry, 38,* 179–186.

Dawson, S., Frey, K., Self, J., Panagiotides, D., Hessl, D., Yamada, E., & Rinaldi, J. (1999). Frontal brain electrical activity in infants of depressed and nondepressed mothers: Relation to variations in infant behavior. *Development and Psychopathology, 11,* 589–605.

Dawson, S., Grofer-Klinger, L., Panagiotides, H., Hilld, D., Spieker, S., & Frey, K. (1992). Infants of mothers with depressive symptoms: Electrophysiological and behavioral findings related to attachment status. *Development and Psychopathology, 4,* 67–80.

Dawson, S., Hessl, D., & Frey, K. (1994). Social influences on early developing biological and behavioral systems related to risk for affective disorder. *Development and Psychopathology, 6,* 759–779.

Dawson, S., Panagiotides, H., Klinger, L., & Spieker, S. (1997). Infants of depressed and non-depressed mothers exhibit difference in frontal brain electrical activity during the expression of negative emotions. *Developmental Psychology, 33,* 650–656.

DeCasper, A., & Fifer, W. (1980). On human bonding: Newborns prefer their mothers' voices. *Science, 208,* 1174.

DeCasper, A., & Spence, M. (1986). Prenatal maternal speech influences newborns' perception of speech sounds. *Infant Behavior and Development, 9,* 133–150.

Demos, V., & Kaplan, S. (1986). Motivation and affect reconsidered: Affect biographies of two infants. *Psychoanalysis and Contemporary Thought, 9,* 147–221.

Donovan, W., & Leavitt, L. (1992). Maternal self-efficacy: Illusory control and its effect on susceptibility to learned helplessness. *Child Development, 61,* 1638–1647.

Dukewich, T., Borkowski, J., & Whitman, T. (1996). Adolescent mothers and child abuse potential: An evaluation of risk factors. *Child Abuse and Neglect, 20,* 1031–1047.

Edward, J., & Sanville, J. (1996). *Fostering healing and growth: A psychoanalytic social work approach.* Northvale, NJ: Jason Aronson.

Ekman, P. (1972). Universal and cultural differences in facial expression of emotion. In J. R. Cole (Ed.), *Nebraska symposium on motivation* (Vol. 19, pp. 207–283). Lincoln, NE: University of Nebraska Press.

Ekman, P., & Friesen, W. V. (1975). *Unmasking the face: A guide to recognizing emotions from facial clues.* Englewood Cliffs, NJ: Prentice-Hall.

Ekman, P., & Friesen, W. V. (1978). *Facial action coding system: A technique for the measurement of facial movement.* Palo Alto, CA: Consulting Psychologists Press.

Elkind, D., & Bowen, R. (1979). Imaginary audience behavior in children and adolescencents. *Developmental Psychology, 15,* 38–44.

Elson, M. (1986). *Self psychology in clinical social work.* New York: Norton.

Emde, R. N. (1980). Toward a psychoanalytic theory of affect, I & II. In S. I. Greenspan & G. H. Pollock (Eds.), *The course of life: Psychoanalytic contributions toward understanding personality development. Vol. 1. Infancy and early childhood* (pp. 63–112). Washington, DC: Mental Health Study Center, U.S. Department of Health and Human Services.

Emde, R. N. (1984). Levels of meaning for infant emotions: A biosocial view. In K. Schere & P. Ekman (Eds.), *Approaches to emotion* (pp. 77–107). Hillsdale, NJ: Erlbaum.

Erickson, M. F., Sroufe, L. A., & Egeland, B. (1985). The relation between quality of attachment and behavior problems in preschooling a high-risk sample. *Monographs for Research in Child Development 50* (1–2), 147–166.

Erikson, E. H. (1968). *Identity: Youth and Crisis.* NY: W. W. Norton & Company.

Field, T. (1995). Infants of depressed mothers. *Infant behavior and development, 18,* 1–13.

Field, T., Estroff, D., Yando, R., del Valle, C., Malphurs, J., & Hart, S. (1996). "Depressed" mothers' perceptions of infant vulnerability are related to later development. *Child Psychiatry and Human Development, 27*(1), 43–53.

Field, T., Woodson, R., Greenberg, R., & Cohen, D. (1982). Discrimination and imitation of facial expressions by neonates. *Science, 218,* 179–181.

Flanagan, P., McGrath, M., Meyer, E., & Garcia-Coll, C. (1995). Adolescent development and transitions to motherhood. *Pediatrics, 96,* 273–277.

Fonagy, P. (1998). An attachment theory approach to treatment of the difficult patient. *Bulletin of the Menninger Clinic, 62,* 147–169.

Fonagy, P., Gergely, G., Jurist, E. L., & Target, M. (2002). *Affect regulation, mentalization and the development of the self.* New York: Other Press.

Fonagy, P., Steele, H., Moran, G., Steele, M., & Higgit, A. (1991). The capacity for understanding mental states: The reflective self in parent and child and its significance for security of attachment. *Infant Mental Health Journal, 13,* 200–217.

Fonagy, P., Steele, M., Steele, H., Leigh, T., Kennedy, R., Mattoon, G., & Target, M. (1995). The predictive validity of Mary Main's Adult Attachment Interview: A psychoanalytic and developmental perspective on the transgenerational transmission of attachment and borderline states. In S. Goldberg, R. Muir, & J. Kerr (Eds.), *Attachment theory: Social, developmental and clinical perspectives* (pp. 233–278). Hillsdale, NJ: Analytic Press.

Fonagy, P., & Target, J. (1998). Mentalization and the changing aims of child psychoanalysis. *Psychoanalytic Dialogues, 8,* 87–114.

Fraiberg, S. (1980). *Clinical studies in infant mental health: The first year of life.* New York: Basic Books.

Fraiberg, S. (1987). The clinical dimensions of baby games. In L. Fraiberg (Ed.), *Selected writings of Selma Fraiberg* (pp. 362–387). Columbus: Ottio University Press.

Fraiberg, S., Adelson, E., & Shapiro, V. (1975). Ghosts in the nursery: A psychoanalytic approach to the problems of impaired infant–mother relationships. *Journal of the American Academy of Child Psychiatry, 14,* 387–422.

Fraser, M. (1997). *Risk and resilience in childhood: An ecological perspective.* Washington, DC: NASW Press.

Frattaroli, E. (2001). *Healing the soul in the age of the brain: Becoming conscious in an unconscious world.* New York: Viking.

Freud, A. (1946). *The ego and the mechanisms of defense.* New York: International Universities Press. (Original work published 1936)

Freud, A., & Burlingham, D. (1944). *Infants without families: The case for and against residential nurseries.* New York: International Universities Press.

Freud, S. (1953). On narcissism: An introduction. In J. Strachey (Ed. & Trans.), *The standard edition of the complete psychological works of Sigmund Freud* (Vol. 14, pp. 73–102). London: Hogarth Press. (Original work published 1914)

Freud, S. (1953). Three essays on the theory of sexuality. In J. Strachey (Ed. & Trans.), *The standard edition of the complete psychological works of Sigmund Freud* (Vol. 7, pp. 130–231). London: Hogarth Press. (Original work published 1905)

Freud, S. (1954). Inhibitions, symptoms and anxiety. In J. Strachey (Ed. & Trans.), *The standard edition of the complete psychological works of Sigmund Freud* (Vol. 20, pp. 87–172). London: Hogarth Press, 1959. (Original work published 1926)

Freud, S. (1961). The economic problem of masochism. In J. Strachey (Ed. & Trans.), *The standard edition of the complete psychological works of Sigmund Freud* (Vol. 19, pp. 159–170). London: Hogarth Press, 1961. (Original work published 1924)

Freud, S. (1961). The ego and the id. In J. Strachey (Ed. & Trans.), *The standard edition of the complete psychological works of Sigmund Freud* (Vol. 19, pp. 3–66). London: Hogarth Press. (Original work published 1923)

Freud, S. (1963). Anxiety. In J. Strachey (Ed. & Trans.), *The standard edition of the complete psychological works of Sigmund Freud* (Vol. 16, pp. 392–411). London: Hogarth Press. (Original work published 1917)

Freud, S. (1966). Project for a scientific psychology. In J. Strachey (Ed. & Trans.), *The standard edition of the complete psychological works of Sigmund Freud* (Vol. 1, pp. 281–397). London: Hogarth Press. (Original work published 1895)

Freud, S. (1966). Some points for a comparative study of organic and hysterical motor paralyses. In J. Strachey (Ed. & Trans.), *The standard edition of the complete psychological works of Sigmund Freud* (Vol. 1, pp. 160–172). London: Hogarth Press. (Original work published 1893)

Furmark, T., Tillfors, M., Marteindottir, I., Fischer, H., Pissiota, A., Langstrom B., & Fredrikson, M. (2002). Common change in cerebral blood flow in patients with social phobia treated with citalopram or cognitive-behavioral therapy. *Archives of General Psychiatry, 59,* 425–433)

Furstenberg, F., Brooks-Gunn, J., & Levine, J. (1990). The children of teenage mothers: Patterns of early childbearing in two generations. *Family Planning Perspectives, 22,* 54–61.

Gabbard, G. O. (1992). Psychodynamic psychiatry in the decade of the brain. *American Journal of Psychiatry, 149,* 991–998.

Galinsky, E. (1998). Child care caregiver sensitivity and attachment. *Social Development, 7,* 25–36.

Garcia-Coll, C., Hoffman, J., & Oh, W. (1987). The social context of teenage childbearing: Effects on the infant's caregiving environment. *Journal of Youth and Adolescence, 16,* 345–360.

George, C., Kaplan, N., & Main, M. (1996). *The adult attachment interview,* unpublished manuscript. Department of Psychology: University of California at Berkley.

Germain, C. B., & Gitterman, A. (1980). *The life model of social work practice.* New York: Columbia University Press.

Goldstein, E. G. (2001). *Object relations theory and self psychology in social work practice.* New York: Free Press.

Goldstein, J., & Goldstein, S. (1996). "Put yourself in the skin of the child," she said. *Psychoanalytic Study of the Child, 51,* 46–55.

Goleman, D. (1995). *Emotional intelligence.* New York: Bantam Books.

Gottlieb, R. M. (2003). Psychosomatic medicine: The divergent legacies of Freud and Janet. *Journal of the American Psychoanalytic Association, 51,* 857–881.

Graham, M., White, B., Clarke, C., & Adams, S. (2001). Infusing infant mental health practices into front-line caregiving. *Infants and Young Children, 14,* 14–23.

Greatrex, T. (2002). Projective identification: How does it work? *Neuropsychoanalysis, 4,* 187–197.

Greenberg, J. R., & Mitchell, S. A. (1983). *Object relations in psychoanalytic theory.* Cambridge, MA: Harvard University Press.

Greenough, W., Black, J., Klintsova, A., Bates, K., Weiler, I. (1999). Experience and plasticity in brain structure: Possible implications of basic research findings for developmental disorders. In Fletcher, J. and Broman, S. (Eds.), *The changing nervous system: Neurobehavioral consequences of early brain disorders* (pp. 51–70). London: Oxford University Press.

Greenough, W. T., Black, J. E., & Wallace, C. (1987). Experience and brain development. *Child Development, 58,* 539–559.

Greenspan, S., & Porges, S. (1984). Psychopathology in infancy and early childhood: Clinical perspectives on the organization of sensory and affective-thematic experience. *Child Development, 55,* 49–71.

Gross, J. J. (1998). *The emerging field of emotion regulation: An integrative review*. New York: Guilford Press.

Gunnar, M., Morison, S., Chisholm, K., & Schuder, M. (2001). Long-term effects of institutional rearing on cortisol levels in adopted Romanian children. *Development & Psychopathology 13*(3), 611–628.

Gunnar, M. (1998). Quality of care and the buffering of stress physiology: Its potential role in protecting the developing human brain. *Newsletter of the Infant Mental Health Promotion Project, 21*, 4–7.

Gunnar, M. (2000). Early adversity and the development of stress reactivity and regulation. In Nelson, C. (Ed.), *The effects of adversity on neurobehavioral, development: Minnesota symposium on child psychology* (31, pp. 163–200). Mahwah, NJ: Lawrence Erlbaum.

Gunnar, M. (2001). Effects of early deprivation. In Nelson, C. and Luciana, M. (Eds.). *Handbook of developmental cognitive neuroscience* (pp. 617–629). Cambridge, MA: MIT Press.

Gunnar, M., Brodersen, L., Nachmias, M., Buss, K., and Rigatuso, R. (1996). Stress reactivity and attachment security. *Developmental Psychobiology, 29*, 191–204.

Gunnar, M., Bruce, J. and Grotevant, H. (2000). International adoption of institutionally reared children: Research and policy. *Development and Psychopathology, 12*(4), 677–693.

Harlow, H. (1958). The nature of love. *American Psychologist, 13*, 673–685.

Hart, S., Gunnar, M., & Cicchetti, D. (1996). Altered neuroendocrine activity in maltreated children related to symptoms of depression. *Development and Psychopathology, 8*(1), 201–214.

Hatcher, S. (1976). Understanding adolescent pregnancy and abortion. *Primary Care, 3*, 407–425.

Hebb, D. O. (1949). *The organization of behavior: A neuropsychological theory*. New York: Wiley.

Hofer, M. (1995). Hidden regulators: Implications for a new understanding of attachment, separation and loss. In S. Goldberg, R. Muir, & J. Kerr (Eds.), *Attachment theory: Social, developmental and clinical perspectives* (pp. 580–592). Hillsdale, NJ: Analytic Press.

Hofferth, S. (1987). The effects of programs and policies on adolescent pregnancy and childbearing. In C. Hayes (Ed.), *Risking the future* (Vol. 1, pp. 123–140). Washington, DC: National Academy Press.

Hudson, C. G. (2000). At the edge of chaos: A new paradigm for social work? *Journal of Social Work Education, 36*, 215–230.

Hughes, S., Catania, P., Derevensky, J., & Dongier, S. (1997). The relationship between maternal psychiatric disorder and very young children's coping behavior. *Infant Mental Health Journal, 18*(1), 58–75.

Imre, R. M. (1982). *Knowing and caring: Philosophical issues in social work*. New York: University Press of America.

Ito, Y., Teicher, M., Glod, C., & Ackerman, E. (1998). Aberrant cortical development in abused children: A quantitative EEG study. *Journal of Neuropsychiatry and Clinical Neuroscience, 10*, 293–307.

Izard, C. E. (1971). *The face of emotion*. New York: Appleton-Century-Crofts.

Jeannerod, M., Arbib, M. A., Rizzolatti, G., & Sakata, H. (1995). Grasping objects: The cortical mechanism of visuomotor transformation. *Trends in Neuroscience, 18*, 314–320.

Josselson, R. (1987). *Finding herself: Pathways to identity development in women.* San Francisco: Jossey-Bass.

Kaler, S., & Freeman, B. J. (1994). Analysis of enviromnental deprivation: Cognitive and social development in Romanian orphanages. *Journal of Child Psychiatry and Allied Disciplines, 35*(4), 769–781.

Kissman, K., & Shapiro, J. (1990). The composites of social support and well-being among adolescent mothers. *International Journal of Adolescence and Youth, 2,* 165–173.

Klaus, M., & Kennel, J. (1998). Bonding: recent observations that alter perinatal care. *Perinatal Review, 19*(1), 4–12.

Kohut, H. (1971). *The analysis of the self.* New York: International Universities Press.

Kohut, H. (1977). *The restoration of the self.* New York: International Universities Press.

Kroger, J. (2000). *Identity development: Adolescence through adulthood.* Thousand Oaks, CA: Sage Publications.

Kroger, J. (2000). *Identity development: Adolescence through adulthood.* Newbury Park, CA: Sage.

Landy, S. (1984). The individuality of teenage mothers and its implications for intervention strategies. *Journal of Adolescence, 7,* 171–290.

Lazarus, R. S. (1991). *Emotion and adaptation.* New York: Oxford University Press.

LeDoux, J. (2000). Cognitive-emotional interactions: Listen to the brain. In R. D. Lane & L. Nadel (Eds.), *Cognitive neuroscience of emotion* (pp. 129–155). New York: Oxford University Press.

LeDoux, J. (1996). *The emotional brain: The mysterious underpinnings of emotional life.* New York: Touchstone.

LeDoux, J. (2002). *Synaptic self: How our brains become who we are.* New York: Penguin Books.

Lewis, M. (1992). Individual differences in the response to stress. *Pediatrics, 3,* 487–490.

Lieberman, A., & Pawl, J. (1990). Disorders of attachment and secure base behavior in the second year of life: Conceptual issues and clinical intervention. In M. Greenberg, D. Cicchetti, & E. Cummings (Eds.), *Attachment in the preschool years* (pp. 375–398). Chicago: University of Chicago Press.

Lieberman, A., Wieder, S., & Fenichel, E. (1997). *The DC:0-3 casebook: A guide to the use of 0 to 3's Diagnostic Classification of Mental Health and Developmental Disorders of Infancy and Early Childhood in Assessment and Treatment Planning.* Washington DC: Zero to Three/National Center for Infants, Toddlers and Families.

Lieberman, A. F., & Zeanah, C. H. (1995). Disorders of attachment in infancy. *Infant Psychiatry, 4,* 571–587.

Linehan, M. M. (1993). *Cognitive–behavioral treatment of borderline personality disorder.* New York: Guilford Press.

Lott, D. (1998). Brain development, attachment and impact on psychic vulnerability. *Psychiatric Times, 15,* 1–5.

Lundy, B., Field, T., Pickens, J., & Cigales, M. (1997). Vocal and facial expression matching in infants of mothers with depressive symptoms. *Infant Mental Health Journal, 18,* 265–273.

Lyons-Ruth, K., Bronfman, E., & Parsons, E. (1999). Maternal frightened, frightening or atypical behavior and disorganized attachment patterns. *Monographs of the Society for Research in Child Development, 64,* 67–96.

MacFarlane, A. (1975). Olfaction in the development of social preferences in the human neonate. In M. Hofer (Ed.), *Parent–infant interaction* (pp. 103–117). Amsterdam: Elsevier.

Mahler, M. S., Pine, F., & Bergman, A. (1975). *The psychological birth of the human infant*. New York: Basic Books.

Main, M., & Goldwyn, R. (1991). *Adult attachment classification system, Version 5*. Berkeley, CA: University of California, Berkeley.

Markus, H., & Nurius, P. (1986). Possible Selves. *American Psychologist, 41*, 954–969.

Maxmen, J. S., & Ward, N. G. (1995). *Essential psychopathology and its treatment* (2nd ed.). New York: Norton.

McEwen, B. (2001). Introduction to Part II: Beyond Nature/Nurture: Genes, Brain and Behavior. *ANN NY AcadSci, 935*, 39–41.

McGoldrick, M., & Gerson, R. (1989). Genograms and the family life cycle. In B. Carter & M. McGoldrick (Eds.), *The changing family life cycle: A framework for family therapy* (2nd ed., pp. 164–189). Needham Heights, MA: Allyn & Bacon.

Meritesacker, B., Bade, U., Haverkock, A., & Pauli-Pott, U. (2004). Predicting maternal reactivity/sensitivity: The role of infant emotionality, maternal depressiveness/anxiety and social support. *Infant Mental Health Journal, 25*(1), 47–61.

Miller, C., Miceli, P., Whitman, T., & Borkowski, J. (1996). Cognitive readiness to parent and intellectural–emotional development in children of adolescent mothers. *Developmental Psychology, 32*, 533–541.

Mitchell, S. (1988). *Relational concepts in psychoanalysis*. Cambridge, MA: Harvard University Press.

Moore, B. E., & Fine, B. D. (Eds.). (1990). *Psychoanalytic terms and concepts*. New Haven, CT: Yale University Press.

Moore, K., & Snyder, N. (1990). *Cognitive development among the children of adolescent mothers*. Washington, DC: Child Trends.

Muir, E. (1992). Watching, waiting and wondering: Applying psychoanalytic principles to mother–infant intervention. *Infant Mental Health Journal, 13*, 319–328.

Nachmias, M., Gunnar, M., Mangesldorf, S., Parritz, R., & Buss, K. (1996). Behavioral inhibition and stress reactivity: Moderating role of attachment security. *Child Development, 67*, 508–522.

Nath, P., Borkowski, J., Whitman, T., & Schellenbach, C. (1991). Understanding adolescent parenting: The dimensions and functions of social support. *Family Relations, 40*, 411–419.

National Clearinghouse on Child Abuse and Neglect. (1993). Child abuse: Intervention and treatment issues. Washington, DC: Department of Health and Human Services.

Nelson, C. A., & Bloom, F. E. (1997). Child development and neuroscience. *Child Development, 68*(5), 970–987.

Nelson, C. A., & Bloom, F. E. (1997). Child development and neuroscience. *Child neurobiological and development basis for psychotherapeutic intervention*.

Newman, B. M., & Newman, P. R. (2003). *Development through life: A psychosocial approach* (8th ed.). Belmont, CA: Wadsworth/Thomson Learning.

Noshpitz, J., & King, R. (1991). *Pathways of growth: Essentials of child psychiatry, Vol. 1. Normal Development*. New York: Wiley.

Olds, D., Eckenrode, J., & Henderson, C. (1997). Long-term effects of home visitation on maternal life course and child abuse and neglect. *Journal of the American Medical Association, 278*, 637–643.

Osofsky, J., Eberhart-Wright, A., Ware, L., & Hann, D. (1992). Children of adolescent mothers: A group at risk for psychopathology. *Infant Mental Health Journal, 13*(2), 119–131.

Page, T. (2000). The attachment partnership as conceptual base for exploring the impact of child maltreatment. *Child and Adolescent Social Work, 16*(6), 419–437.

Pally, R. (2000). *The mind–brain relationship.* London: Karnac Books.

Panksepp, J. (1998). *Affective neuroscience: The foundations of human and animal emotions.* New York: Oxford University Press.

Paret, I., & Shapiro, V. (1998). The splintered holding environment and the vulnerable ego: A case study. *Psychoanalytic Study of the Child, 53,* 300–324.

Parlakian, R. (2001). *Look, Listen and Learn: Reflective Supervision and Relationship-based Work.* Washington, DC: Zero-to-Three Press.

Perlman, H. H. (1957). *Social casework: A problem-solving process.* Chicago: University of Chicago Press.

Perlman, H. H. (1979). *Relationship, the heart of helping people.* Chicago: University of Chicago Press.

Perrett, D. I., Rolls, E. T., & Cann, W. (1982). Visual neurons responsive to faces in the monkey temporal cortex. *Experimental Brain Research, 47,* 329–342.

Perry, B. (1995). Incubated in terror: Neurodevelopmental factors in the cycle of violence. In J. D. Osofsky (Ed.), *Children, youth and violence: Searching for solutions* (pp. 271–291). New York: Guilford Press.

Perry, B., Pollard, R., Blakley, T., Baker, W., & Vigilante, D. (1995). Childhood trauma, the neurobiology of adaptation, and "use-dependent" development of the brain: How "states" become "traits." *Infant Mental Health Journal, 16*(4), 271–289.

Phillips, D., Howes, C. and Whitebook, M. (2002). The social policy context of child care: Effects on quality. In D'Augelli, A. and Revenson, T. (Eds.), *A quarter century of community psychology: Readings from the American Journal of Community Psychology* (pp. 367–393). New York: Kluwer Academic/Plenum Publishers.

Pliszka, S. R. (2003). *Neuroscience for the mental health clinician.* New York: Guilford Press.

Pollak, S., Cicchetti, D., Klorman, R., & Brumaghim, J. (1997). Cognitive brain ERP and emotional processing in maltreated children. *Child Development, 68*(5), 773–383.

Ponirakis, A., Susman, E., & Stifter, C. (1999). Negative emotionality and cortisol during adolescent pregnancy and its effects on infant health and autonomic nervous system reactivity. *Developmental Psychobiology, 33,* 163–174.

Pope, S., Whiteside, L., Brooks-Gunn, J., Kelleher, K., Rickert, V., Bradley, R., & Casey, P. (1993). Low-birthweight infants born to adolescent mothers: Effects of coresidency with grandmother on child development. *Journal of the American Medical Association, 269,* 1396–1400.

Post, R., Weiss, S., Smith, M., & Li, H. (1997). Kindling versus quenching: Implications for the evolution and treatment of posttraumatic stress disorder. *Annals of the New York Academy of Sciences, 821,* 285–295.

Pulver, S. E. (2003). On the astonishing clinical irrelevance of neuroscience. *Journal of the American Psychoanalytic Association, 51,* 755–772.

Radin, N., Oyserman, D., & Benn, R. (1990, April). *Grandfather influence on the young children of teenage mothers.* Paper presented at the biennial meeting of the Society for Research on Child Development, Kansas City, MO.

Reid, W. J. (2001). The scientific and empirical foundations of clinical social work. In H. E. Briggs & K. Corcoran (Eds.), *Social work practice: Treating common client problems* (pp. 37–53). Chicago: Lyceum.

Roumell, N., Wille, D., Abramson, L., & Delaney, V. (1997). Facial expressivity to acute pain in cocaine exposed toddlers. *Infant Mental Health Journal, 18*, 274–281.

Russel, C. S. (1980). Unscheduled parenthood: Transitions to "parent" for the teenager. *Journal of Social Issues, 365*, 45–63.

Saari, C. (2002). *The environment: Its role in psychosocial functioning and psychotherapy*. New York: Columbia University Press.

Sadler, L., & Catrone, C. (1983). The adolescent parent: A dual developmental crisis. *Journal of Adolescent Health Care, 4*, 100–105.

Sameroff, A., & Fiese, B. (1990). Transactional regulation and emotion. In Shonkoff, J., & Meisels, S. (Eds.), *Handbook of Early Childhood Intervention* (pp. 119–149). NY: Cambridge University Press.

Sanville, J. (1991). *The playground of psychoanalytic therapy*. Hillsdale, NJ: Analytic Press.

Schacter, D. L. (1996). *Searching for memory: The brain, the mind, and the past*. New York: Basic Books.

Schamess, G. (1991). Toward an understanding of the etiology and treatment of psychological dysfunction among single teenage mothers. *Smith College School of Social Work, 60*, 143–175.

Schore, A. N. (1994). *Affect regulation and the origin of the self: The neurobiology of emotional development*. Hillsdale, NJ: Erlbaum.

Schore, A. N. (1996). The experience-dependent maturation of a regulatory system in the orbital prefrontal cortex and the origins of developmental psychopathology. *Development and Psychopathology, 8*, 59–87.

Schore, A. N. (1997a). A century after Freud's *Project*: Is a rapprochement between psychoanalysis and neurobiology at hand? *Journal of American Psychoanalytic Association, 45*, 809–840.

Schore, A. N. (1997b). Interdisciplinary developmental research as a source of clinical models. In M. Moskowitz, C. Monk, C.Kaye, & S. Ellman (Eds.), *The neurobiological and developmental basis for psychotherapeutic intervention* (pp. 1–71). Northvale, NJ: Jason Aronson.

Schore, A. N. (2000). Attachment and the regulation of the right brain. *Attachment and Human Development, 2*, 23–47.

Schore, A. N. (2001). Effects of a secure attachment relationship on right brain development, affect regulation and infant mental health. *Infant Mental Health Journal, 22*, 7–66.

Schore, A. N. (2003a). *Affect dysregulation and disorders of the self*. New York: Norton.

Schore, A. N. (2003b). *Affect regulation and the repair of the self*. New York: Norton.

Schwartz, J. M., & Begley, S. (2002). *The mind and the brain: Neuroplasticity and the power of mental force*. New York: Regan Books.

Schwartz, J. M., Stoessel, P. W., Baxter, L. R., Jr., Martin, K. M., & Phelps, M. E. (1996). Systematic cerebral glucose metabolic rate changes after successful behavior modification treatment of obsessive–compulsive disorder. *Archives of General Psychiatry, 53*, 109–113.

Seitz, V., & Apfel, N. (1993). Adolescent mothers and repeated childbearing: Effects of a school-based intervention program. *American Journal of Orthopsychiatry, 63*(4), 572–581.

Selkoe, D. (1998). Cellular-production of amyloid beta-protein: A direct route to the mechanism and treatment of Alzheimer's disease. In Marhal, F. (Ed.), *Neurobiology of primary dementia* (pp. 43–51). New York: Association for Research in Nervous and Mental Disease/American Psychiatric Association.

Seinfeld, J. (1991). *The empty core: An object relations approach to psychotherapy of the schizoid personality.* Hillsdale, NJ: Jason Aronson.

Shapiro, J. (2002). The developmental context of adolescent motherhood. In Farber, N., *Adolescent Pregnancy: Policy and Prevention Services* (pp. 38–52). NY: Springer.

Shapiro, J., & Applegate, J. (2000). The neurobiology of affect regulation: Implications for clinical social work. *Clinical Social Work, 28,* 1–28.

Shapiro, J., & Mangelsdorf, S. (1994). The determinants of parenting competence in adolescent mothers. *Journal of Youth and Adolescence, 23*(6), 621–641.

Shapiro, V., Shapiro, J., & Paret, I. (2001). *Complex adoption and assisted reproductive technology: A developmental approach to clinical practice.* New York: Guilford Press.

Shields, A., & Cicchetti, D. (2001). Parental maltreatment and emotion dysregulation as risk factors for bullying and victimization in middle childhood. *Journal of Clinical Child Psychology, 30*(3), 349–363.

Shonkoff, J., & Phillips, D. (Eds.). (2000). *From neurons to neighborhoods: The science of early childhood development.* Washington, DC: National Academy Press.

Siegel, D. J. (1998). The developing mind: Toward a neurobiology of interpersonal experience. *The Signal: Newsletter of the World Association for Infant, 6,* 1–10.

Siegel, D. J. (1999). *The developing mind: Toward a neurobiology of interpersonal experience.* New York: Guilford Press.

Slade, A. (2002). Keeping the baby in mind: A critical factor in perinatal mental healh. In Special Issue on Perinatal Mental Health. *Zero to Three,* June/July, 521–529.

Solms, M., & Turnbull, O. (2002). *The brain and the inner world: An introduction to the neuroscience of subjective experience.* New York: Other Press.

Solomon, J., & George, C. (1999). *Attachment disorganization.* New York: Guilford Press.

Spezzano, C. (1993). *Affect in psychoanalysis: A clinical synthesis.* Hillsdale, NJ: Analytic Press.

Spitz, R., & Wolf, K. (1946). Anaclitic depression: An inquiry into the genesis of psychiatric conditions in early childhood, II. *Psychoanalytic Study of the Child, 2,* 313–342.

Sroufe, L., Egeland, B., & Kreutzer, T. (1990). The fate of early experience following developmental change: Longitudinal approaches to understanding adaptation in childhood. *Child Development, 61,* 1363–1373.

Sroufe, L. A. (2000). Early relationships and the development of children. *Infant Mental Health Journal, 21*(1–2), 67–74.

Steele, H., Steele, M., & Fonagy, P. (1996). Associations among attachment classifications of mothers, fathers and their infants. *Child Development, 67*(2), 541–555.

Steele, H., Steele, M., Croft, C., & Fonagy, P. (1999). Infant–mother attachment at one year predicts children's understanding of mixed emotions at six years. *Social Development, 8,* 161–178.

Stein, M., Hanna, C., Koverola, C., & Torchia, M. (1997). Structural brain changes in PTSD: Does trauma alter neuroanatomy? *Annals of the New York Academy of Sciences, 821,* 76–82.

Stein, M., Hanna, C., Vaerum, V., & Koverola, C. (1999). Memory functioning in adult women traumatized by childhood sexual abuse. *Journal of Traumatic Stress, 12*(3), 527–534.

Stern, D. N. (1985). *The interpersonal world of the infant: A view from psychoanalysis and developmental psychology.* New York: Basic Books.

Stolorow, R. D., Atwood, G. E., & Brandchaft, B. (1994). *The intersubjective perspective.* Northvale, NJ: Jason Aronson.

Teicher, M. H. (2002, March). The neurobiology of child abuse. *Scientific American,* 68–75.

Tomkins, S. S. (1962). *Affect, imagery, consciousness. Vol I. The positive affects.* New York: Springer.

Tomkins, S. S. (1963). *Affect, imagery, consciousness. Vol. II. The negative affects.* New York: Springer.

Tomkins, S. S. (1995). What and where are the primary affects? Some evidence for a theory. In E.V. Demos (Ed.), *Exploring affect: The selected writings of Silvan S. Tomkins* (pp. 217–262). Cambridge, UK: Cambridge University Press. (Original work published 1964)

Trevarthen, C., & Aitken, K. (1994). Brain development, infant communication and empathy disorders: Intrinsic factors in child mental health. *Development and Psychopathology, 6,* 597–633.

Tronick, E. (1989). Emotions and emotional communication in infants. *American Psychologist, 44,* 112–119.

Tronick, E., Als, H., Adamson, L., Wise, S., & Brazelton, T. B. (1978). The infant's response to entrapment between contradictory messages in face-to-face interaction. *Journal of the American Academy of Child and Adolescent Psychiatry, 17,* 1–13.

Tronick, E., & Beeghly, M. (1992). Effects of prenatal exposure to cocaine on newborn behavior and development: A critical review. *OSAP Prevention Monograph, 11,* 25–48.

Tronick, E., & Weinberg, M. (1998). The impact of maternal psychiatric illness on infant development. *Journal of Clinical Psychiatry, 59,* 53–61.

Tyson, P. (2002). The challenges of psychoanalytic developmental theory. *Journal of the American Psychoanalytic Association, 50,* 19–52.

von Bertalanffy, L. (1968). *General systems theory: Foundation, development, applications.* New York: Braziller.

Ward, M., Botyanski, N., Plunkett, S., & Carlson, E. (1991, April). *The concurrent and predictive validity of the AAI for adolescent mothers.* Paper presented at the biennial meeting of the Society for Research in Child Development, Seattle, WA.

Ward, M., & Carlson, E. (1995). Associations among adult attachment representations, maternal sensitivity and infant-mother attachment in a sample of adolescent mothers. *Child Development, 66,* 69–79.

Watson, J. S. (1972). Smiling, cooing, and "the game." *Merrill–Palmer Quarterly, 18,* 323–339.

Weatherston, D., & Baltman, K. (1995). *Assessing the parent-infant relationship: Observable strengths and risks.* Detroit, MI: Merrill-Palmer Institute, Wayne State University.

Weatherston, D. (2000, October/November). The infant mental health specialist. *Zero to Three,* pp. 46–83.

Webb, N.B. (1996). *Social work practice with children*. New York: Guilford Press.

Westen, D., & Gabbard, G. L. (2002). Developments in cognitive neuroscience: II. Implications for theories of transference. *Journal of the American Psychoanalytic Association, 50*, 99–134.

Wheeler, R. E., Davidson, R. J., & Tomarken, A. J. (1993). Frontal brain asymmetry and emotional reactivity. A biological substrate of affective style. *Psychophysiology, 30*, 82–89.

Whitman, T., Borkowski, J., Schellenbach, C., & Nath, P. (1987). Predicting and understanding developmental delay of children of adolescent mothers: A multi-dimensional approach. *American Journal of Mental Deficiency, 92*, 40–56.

Winnicott, D. W. (1965a). The capacity to be alone. In *The maturational processes and the facilitating environment* (pp. 29–36). Madison, CT: International Universities Press. (Original work published 1958)

Winnicott, D. W. (1965b). Ego distortion in terms of true and false self. In *The maturational processes and the facilitating environment* (pp. 140–152). Madison, CT: International Universities Press. (Original work published 1960)

Winnicott, D. W. (1965c). Ego integration in child development. In *The maturational processes and the facilitating environment* (pp. 56–63). Madison, CT: International Universities Press. (Original work published 1962)

Winnicott, D. W. (1965d). *The maturational processes and the facilitating environment*. Madison, CT: International Universities Press.

Winnicott, D. W. (1971). Mirror-role of mother and family in child development. In *Playing and reality* (pp. 111–118). London: Tavistock.

Winnicott, D. W. (1975). *Through paediatrics to psycho-analysis*. New York: Basic Books.

Zajonc, R. B. (1984). The interaction of affect and cognition. In K. R. Scherer & P. Ekman (Eds.), *Approaches to emotion* (pp. 239–246). Hillsdale, NJ: Erlbaum.

Zero to Three: National Center for Infants, Toddlers and Families (1994). *Diagnostic classification of mental health and developmental disorders of infancy and early childhood*. Washington, DC: Zero to Three.

Zuckerman, B. (1997, May). *Brain development in infants and young children*. Paper presented at the Conference on Early Childhood Education. Woodrow Wilson School of Public Policy, Princeton University, Princeton, NJ.

INDEX

233